Treating PTSD

TREATMENT MANUALS FOR PRACTITIONERS
David H. Barlow, *Editor*

Treating PTSD
Cognitive–Behavioral Strategies

Edited by

DAVID W. FOY

Fuller Theological Seminary
West Los Angeles Veterans Affairs Medical Center,
Brentwood Division

Series Editor's Note by David H. Barlow

THE GUILFORD PRESS
New York   London

© 1992 The Guilford Press
A Division of Guilford Publications, Inc.
72 Spring Street, New York, NY 10012

Printed in the United States of America

This book is printed on acid-free paper.

Last digit is print number: 9   8   7   6   5   4   3

Library of Congress Cataloging-in-Publication Data

Treating PTSD: cognitive–behavioral strategies / edited by David W.
    Foy.
        p.   cm. — (Treatment manuals for practitioners)
    Includes bibliographical references and index.
        ISBN 0-89862-209-3 (hard). — ISBN 0-89862-220-4 (pbk.)
    1. Post-traumatic stress disorder — Treatment. 2. Cognitive
therapy.   I. Foy, David W., 1944–   . II. Series: Treatment
manuals for practitioners.
    [DNLM: 1. Behavior Therapy. 2. Cognitive Therapy. 3. Stress
Disorders, Post-Traumatic — therapy.   WM 170 T784]
RC552.P67T765 1992
616.85'21 — dc20
DNLM/DLC
for Library of Congress   92-1463
                                                                  CIP

Contributors

Edward M. Carroll, PhD, West Los Angeles Department of Veterans Affairs Medical Center, Brentwood Division, Los Angeles, California; Department of Psychology, University of California at Los Angeles, Los Angeles, California

Mary Ann Dutton, PhD, Family Violence Program, School of Psychology, Nova University, Fort Lauderdale, Florida

David W. Foy, PhD, Graduate School of Psychology, Fuller Theological Seminary, Pasadena, California; West Los Angeles Department of Veterans Affairs Medical Center, Brentwood Division, Los Angeles, California

Julie A. Lipovsky, PhD, Crime Victims Research and Treatment Center, Department of Psychiatry and Behavioral Sciences, Medical University of South Carolina, Charleston, South Carolina

Tamara Newton, MA, Crime Victims Research and Treatment Center, Department of Psychiatry and Behavioral Sciences, Medical University of South Carolina, Charleston, South Carolina

Heidi S. Resnick, PhD, Crime Victims Research and Treatment Center, Department of Psychiatry and Behavioral Sciences, Medical University of South Carolina, Charleston, South Carolina

R. Carl Sipprelle, PhD, Department of Veterans Affairs Medical Center, Sepulveda, California

Acknowledgments

The efforts of a number of individuals were instrumental in compiling and editing this book. Several of my graduate student advisees—Millie Astin, Ned Rodriguez, Suzann Ogland-Hand, Susan Ryan, and Esther Coleman—read and made suggestions for various chapter drafts. My colleague Beverly Haas proofread each chapter as editorial changes were made. Her encouragement and direct contributions to the work were invaluable. Barbara Townsend, my secretary at the Fuller Theological Seminary's Graduate School of Psychology, was helpful in seeing that the many administrative details received appropriate attention.

Several of my fellow traumatologists deserve special mention, because they were constant sources of encouragement and shared the vision that the work was needed. David Hanley, MSW, Lisa Zaidi, PhD, Ed Carroll, PhD, Beth Houskamp, PhD, and Fred Gusman, MSW, helped in this way and also made substantive editorial suggestions. Greg Versen, MSW, and Haig Kojian, PhD, made helpful suggestions for the introductory chapter.

Fuller Theological Seminary granted the necessary sabbatical leave for much of the work to be accomplished, and I thank the Dean and my colleagues from the Graduate School of Psychology for sparing me while this work was in progress.

Most of all I am indebted to my children, Patrick, Danny, Lizzy, and Ben, and my wife, Patty, for providing ongoing encouragement and making the necessary sacrifices so that the work could be completed. It is to them, and to the many survivors whose personal stories of trauma and courage provided the clinical material, that this book is dedicated.

DAVID W. FOY

Series Editor's Note

Few problems have burst upon the international scene with the force of post-traumatic stress disorder (PTSD). Only slightly over 10 years ago, the majority of psychopathologists and nosologists doubted that such a disorder existed. Since that time, recognition of the extraordinary prevalence of trauma-related psychopathology has led to marked changes in our approaches to these problems.

As we have learned more about the debilitating effects of trauma and the chronic nature of many reactions to severe trauma, treatment programs and centers have sprung up around the world to deal with the myriad of problems resulting from war, natural disasters, and personal abuse. Unfortunately, the development of many of these treatment programs has not benefited from examining existing treatment protocols at more established centers. In addition, until very recently, most published work concerned itself with PTSD resulting from war-related trauma; even in this area, however, established treatment protocols have been hard to come by because of the relatively recent development of effective treatment programs.

Now, for the first time, David Foy has collected treatment protocols, most with proven efficacy, in use at established centers. Most importantly, this book presents a "cross-trauma" perspective that highlights the similarities of the treatment of PTSD in a variety of different traumatized populations, such as survivors of combat, child and adult sexual assault, and domestic violence, while at the same time highlighting the very important differences among these groups that require specific tailorings of these treatment protocols. All clinicians working with these populations should find these treatment protocols invaluable in facilitating their own efforts with these unfortunate individuals.

DAVID H. BARLOW
The University at Albany
State University of New York

Preface

This book was written to provide behavioral strategies for assessing and treating survivors of several prevalent types of human-induced psychological trauma. It is intended for graduate students and mental health professionals whose clinical work involves these survivors. It is unique in its "cross-trauma" approach by which familiar behavioral methods— fear extinction, cognitive restructuring, and skills training—are adapted for treating survivors of combat, battering, and sexual assault. While clinical work with each primary trauma population must consider its unique aspects, it is reassuring for clinicians to know that there are basic principles of behavioral assessment and treatment that can be applied across types of survivors.

Toward this objective, respected behaviorally trained clinicians have contributed chapters dealing with survivor groups with whom each has had years of clinical experience. Since combat-related trauma is treated in the Department of Veterans Affairs through two primary routes, R. Carl Sipprelle first describes group methods appropriate for Vet Center applications, while Edward M. Carroll and I add a companion chapter focusing upon individual behavioral methods used in VA Medical Center settings. Mary Ann Dutton distills behavioral principles for treating battered women in shelter or outpatient settings. Heidi S. Resnick and Tamara Newton describe their treatment methods for adult sexual assault survivors, while Julie A. Lipovsky presents behavioral methods used with child survivors.

The behavioral methods presented are intended to inform trauma therapists, regardless of their theoretical orientations, although behaviorally trained clinicians may find it easier to apply the strategies initially. The methods are not presented as mutually exclusive of other psychotherapeutic or pharmacologic approaches. Rather, it is our hope that these principles will be integrated into therapists' current conceptual models for guiding future work.

DAVID W. FOY

Contents

Treating PTSD

1

Introduction and Description of the Disorder

DAVID W. FOY

For more than 10 years, several colleagues in the Los Angeles area and I have focused our primary clinical and research interests upon unsolved problems of assessment and treatment for trauma survivors. Until 1987, these efforts were directed almost exclusively toward combat-related issues presented by Vietnam veterans. At that time, however, a number of my students at the Fuller Theological Seminary's Graduate School of Psychology began to challenge me to think beyond combat trauma. They were interested in the potential applicability of a combat-derived model of post-traumatic stress disorder (PTSD) to issues of other trauma survivors, in the hope that some of the methodological and conceptual gains made in the study of combat could be useful.

Concurrently, some of the former interns with whom I had worked in the Psychology Internship Program at the West Los Angeles Department of Veterans Affairs (VA) Medical Center, Brentwood Division, began to work clinically with other trauma populations, and they related their experiences, both positive and negative, in attempting to adapt their combat-related assessment and treatment methods. At conventions and other professional meetings, I began to meet other colleagues who were making similar adaptations for their clinical work. Often a rapport quickly developed as we shared common experiences in working with our trauma survivors. We all seemed to need to learn from one another; this need was enhanced by the absence of an established body of literature or senior mentors to guide us.

Since the treatment of trauma-related victimization is new as a clinical specialty, well-established guidelines for assessment and treatment are not yet available. Treatment outcome studies upon which to base clinical principles are just now being conducted, and it will be some time before results begin to appear in the literature. In the absence of a clear, empirically derived foundation, there is a pressing need to adapt existing behavioral methods for current clinical work with survivors.

Fortunately, several pioneers have done some significant trail-blazing work with major survivor groups already. It is to this group of fellow behavioral "traumatologists" that I have turned in order to produce this edited work. Contributors have used basic behavioral principles of assessment and treatment to identify key clinical elements for intervention with their particular survivor groups. It is our intention to provide practical clinical tools for therapists who must deal now with trauma survivors while the specialty evolves. Although behavioral principles can be very useful for guiding clinical work, we are not claiming superiority for behavioral treatment of PTSD. Rather, it is our hope that this book will be broadly useful as a reference for professionals already in the field and for graduate courses preparing new mental health professionals to work with trauma survivors.

History and Validity of the Diagnosis

PTSD was introduced into the current diagnostic system in 1980, with the advent of the third edition of the *Diagnostic and Statistical Manual of Mental Disorders* (DSM-III) of the American Psychiatric Association. However, consistent patterns of psychological distress following such sudden traumatic experiences as natural disasters or combat horrors had been described in both professional and popular literature for many years prior to the formal inclusion of PTSD. For example, "shell shock" and "combat fatigue," formulations denoting a presumed organic basis for trauma-related psychological symptoms, were used during the two World Wars. Diagnoses previously used for the disorder included "adjustment reactions" and "pathological" grief responses.

Relative to the conceptualization of other psychological disorders, that of PTSD appears to represent an advance, in that a direct linkage between a known causal agent (a traumatic event) and a resultant syndrome is assumed. Thus, at least in theory, PTSD is an ideal diagnosis; it exceeds the level of simple description of symptoms or predictable pathogenesis that is characteristic of other disorders, for which specific etiology is not yet known. However, there remains considerable controversy about the kinds of traumatic stressors and necessary levels of intensity that would constitute appropriate events for meeting diagnostic criteria. The revised third edition of the *Diagnostic and Statistical Manual* (DSM-III-R; American Psychiatric Association, 1987) does not provide an exhaustive list of events meeting requirements for a bona fide "traumatic stressor" (category A) for a PTSD diagnosis. At this stage, critical elements in defining trauma appear to be that it is "life-threatening," "overwhelming" to almost all human respondents, and "sudden or unexpected" in nature. Accordingly, further empirical study of relationships between presumed traumatic events and predictable distress patterns (PTSD symptoms) is needed before epidemiology of the disorder can be established.

Other issues in validating psychiatric disorders also remain to be settled in the case of PTSD. A diagnosis needs to be different from other diagnoses in the symptom picture presented. Since comorbidity (of substance abuse, depression, and other anxiety disorders) is frequently found in PTSD, its distinctiveness as a separate disorder remains to be convincingly established. In addition, coherence of symptoms, or higher intercorrelations among PTSD symptoms than with symptoms of other disorders, has not yet been empirically demonstrated (Robins, 1990).

Despite these limitations, combat-related PTSD represents a prototype for studying PTSD in other trauma survivors, since it has been studied extensively in recent years. State-of-the-art knowledge about combat-related PTSD is drawn from studies conducted with sound methodology, whereas many studies of other types of trauma are descriptive or anecdotal. Several combat studies with nationally drawn samples have provided consistent findings on two important issues. First, disorder rates have been shown to vary as a function of increasing exposure to distressing combat-related events. Thus, at least for combat-related PTSD, the etiological linkage between trauma exposure and a predictable pattern of psychological distress is well established. Second, PTSD prevalence rates in populations with high combat exposure, in both community and clinical samples, have been reported in the range of 15–50%; this provides an estimate of the relative risk associated with high exposure.

However, determining epidemiology of PTSD in both clinical and community populations has been impeded by methodological limitations of early studies. They have often failed to make adequate distinctions between those subjects who had been exposed to the trauma under study and the remaining subjects who were unexposed. Thus, disorder rates were established without regard to trauma exposure status. However, more recent studies have begun to report trauma exposure rates in the study population as a primary variable of interest, in addition to actual PTSD rates among trauma-exposed individuals (e.g., Breslau, Davis, Andreski, & Peterson, 1991). Thus, prevalence rates for "ecopathology" (environmental adversity through traumatic life events) are now being distinguished from psychopathology rates determined from the proportion of positively diagnosed cases in exposed populations. It is the complex relationship between traumatic ecopathology and increased risk for psychopathology (PTSD cases) that constitutes the unique focus for my colleagues' and my clinical and research activities.

Another critical element that has impeded our understanding of PTSD etiology is the failure to conceptualize trauma exposure in its broader context. Most current studies approach PTSD from the standpoint of studying symptoms presumed to be related to one particular type of trauma exposure. When previous trauma history is examined at all, it is approached as a dichotomous variable determined by simple "yes" or "no" responses to global screening questions about other traumatic experiences.

Recent studies conducted by our Los Angeles-area PTSD research group have addressed a variety of primary trauma populations, including battered women, adult and child sexual assault survivors, gang-involved adolescents, and combat veterans. In the series of studies that have been conducted in each trauma area, we have found that exposure to multiple traumas is the norm rather than the exception. For example, battered women in the clinical samples in our studies also show high rates of childhood physical and sexual abuse and marital rape, in addition to traumatic exposure through being battered by their current intimate partners. Similarly, delinquent youths currently involved in perpetrating violence through gang-related activities show high rates of prior physical abuse; traumatic deaths in their immediate families; and personal victimization through being beaten, shot, or stabbed.

The discovery that, in clinical populations at least, PTSD-positive individuals often have histories of exposures to multiple traumas has led us to change the focus of our research efforts from our original "cross-trauma" perspective to a current "multiple-trauma" view. Consequently, we have become much more interested in studying the "ecopathology" of trauma, as well as its "psychopathology." For the present, at least, we have concentrated upon comprehensive assessment of various types of trauma exposure and related risk for PTSD as a priority for our work.

Knowledge of the Disorder

Ecopathology

Exposure rates for the primary trauma types being addressed in this book vary across clinical and community populations, with clinical samples showing higher rates for these traumatic experiences. Thus, it is important to distinguish between the types of populations sampled when prevalence rates for trauma exposure are being considered. Among the 8.2 million Vietnam-era veterans, 3.14 million (38%) actually experienced combat exposure by virtue of assignment within the hostile fire zone (Jordan et al., 1991). Epidemiology of domestic violence has been the topic of several recent national studies in which approximately 12% of female respondents reported incidents of being battered by their spouses (e.g., Straus & Gelles, 1986).

Sexual assault rates for females have been reported by numerous studies of both community and clinical populations. Two national epidemiology studies, conducted almost 40 years apart, revealed remarkably similar rates for unwanted sexual contact before age 18. In 1953, Kinsey, Pomeroy, Martin, and Gebhard found that 24% of their female respondents reported childhood sexual abuse; a recent study conducted by Finkelhor, Hotaling, Lewis, and Smith (1990) produced a 27% rate for females and a 16% rate for males. In clinical samples, childhood sexual abuse rates are typically much higher. Briere and Runtz (1987) reported a 44% exposure rate in women seeking crisis counseling; in a study of women being evaluated in a medical center psychiatric emergency room, Briere and Zaidi (1989) found that 74% reported a history of childhood sexual abuse. Recent studies on community samples have produced findings for prevalence of completed rape during adulthood in women ranging from 13% to 26% (Kilpatrick & Resnick, in press).

Psychopathology

Disorder rates in exposed individuals vary as a function of the degree of exposure. Our research group's comparisons of PTSD rates in clinical subjects with high versus low exposure consistently show that high exposure is associated with more than twice the risk found for low exposure in combat veterans (e.g., Foy, Resnick, Sipprelle, & Carroll, 1987), adult (Rowan, Rodriguez, Gallers, & Foy, 1990) and child (Koverola, Foy, Heger, & Lytle, 1990) sexual assault survivors and battered women

(Houskamp & Foy, 1991). In these studies, "high exposure" has been defined as personal involvement including both physical injury and a perceived threat to life.

A recent national epidemiology study conducted with a probability sample of veterans in community settings revealed a lifetime PTSD prevalence rate of 30%, with 15.2% of subjects showing a current positive diagnosis (Jordan et al., 1991). In our clinical samples of Vietnam combat veterans receiving services in Los Angeles-area VA Medical Centers, current PTSD-positive diagnostic rates often exceed 50% (Foy et al., 1987). Although studies to establish the prevalence of PTSD in community samples of battered women have not yet been reported, clinical samples of battered women residing in shelters or attending community-based self-help groups assessed by our group have shown PTSD rates of 45% in two successive studies (Astin, Lawrence, Pincus, & Foy, 1990; Houskamp & Foy, 1991).

Studies assessing PTSD in children who have been recently sexually abused show positive diagnostic rates of approximately 50% (Koverola et al., 1990; McLeer, Deblinger, Atkins, Foa, & Ralphe, 1988). In a recent study of a clinical sample of adult survivors of childhood sexual assault, a PTSD rate of 65% was obtained (Rowan et al., 1990). Using nationally drawn community samples, current estimates for PTSD prevalence in adult rape victims show current rates of 13% and lifetime rates of 35% (Kilpatrick & Resnick, in press).

Symptoms

Classic symptom patterns in PTSD consist of intrusive thoughts about the traumatic experience(s) and psychological efforts to avoid reminders or cues related to the trauma. Intrusive thoughts may be observed in the waking state in the form of "flashbacks," or intensely vivid re-enactment experiences in which the original traumatic fear and psychological distress is also reactivated. In addition, intrusion patterns may occur during the sleeping state in the form of thematically related nightmares. Avoidance (or escape) patterns may be observed when trauma victims show discomfort followed by shifting attention away from reminders of their traumatic experiences. Successful efforts to avoid painful reminders by eliminating risk of exposure to them may be learned through negative reinforcement. These patterns of intrusion and avoidance are commonly seen in the natural temporary experience of acute grief following the death of a loved one. However, in the case of PTSD, the process by which grief and other overwhelming emotions are eventually resolved through natural coping seems to have been arrested.

Symptom patterns in PTSD include physiological, cognitive, and behavioral manifestations. Autonomic arousal upon presentation of trauma-related cues is consistently found among approximately two-thirds of PTSD-positive combat veterans (e.g., Blanchard, Kolb, Gerardi, Ryan, & Pallmeyer, 1986). Although other trauma populations have not yet been assessed for physiological reactivity in laboratory analogue situations, hypervigilance, exaggerated startle responses, and panic symptoms are frequently reported by these survivors. Thus, it seems reasonable to expect that physiological arousal to traumatic cues may represent an important feature in these cases as well.

Cognitive distortions indicative of "shattered" life assumptions are also frequently observed (Janoff-Bulman, 1985). Critical assumptions about personal invulnerability, equitability and fairness of life, and personal self-worth may shift radically after traumatic victimization. Extreme self-blame, inability to trust others, and constant fear for personal safety may develop to the extent that survivors are rarely free of the need to monitor their interpersonal and physical environments constantly for signs of danger.

Avoidance of trauma-related cues may come to characterize the lifestyles of survivors who are unable to overcome their immediate trauma crisis reactions. Feared stimuli eliciting escape or avoidance responses may not be limited to the physical environment. Strong negative emotions, such as rage, grief, and intense anxiety or panic, may elicit patterns of responding very similar to the individual's original trauma reactions (re-enactment); they may thereby establish escape or avoidant behaviors in a much wider range of situations.

Conceptual Model of PTSD

From our cognitive–behavioral perspective, assessment and treatment efforts are guided by our PTSD etiological hypothesis (Foy, Osato, Houskamp, & Neumann, in press). The model (Figure 1.1) is interactional in nature, so that both environmental and individual factors are assumed to be necessary for understanding the development and maintenance of PTSD symptoms. In our model, individuals are placed at risk for PTSD when exposure to an overwhelming traumatic stressor occurs. An immediate conditioned emotional reaction is hypothesized as a critical link in the causal chain mechanism leading to acute distress. Whether PTSD subsequently develops is influenced by additional medi-

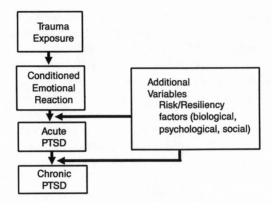

FIGURE 1.1. Conceptual model of PTSD. From "PTSD Etiology" by D. W. Foy, S. S. Osato, B. M. Houskamp, and D. A. Neumann, in press, in P. A. Saigh (Ed.), *Posttraumatic Stress Disorder: Behavioral Assessment and Treatment*, Elmsford, NY: Maxwell Press. Copyright by Maxwell Press. Reprinted by permission.

ating variables from the biological, psychological, and social domains. The model draws from existing formulations (Foa & Kozak, 1986; Kolb, 1988), but presents an advantage: It can account also for the failure to develop PTSD following extreme trauma exposure, through the interaction of mediating variables.

Mediating variables may interact with the primary etiological agent (traumatic event) through several possible routes. First, the presence of an additional factor may place the individual at greater risk for developing PTSD by functioning as a "vulnerability" factor. In this case, the mediating variable has no direct effect by producing distress independently, but its presence interacts with the effects of traumatic experience to heighten reactivity. A mediating factor producing the reverse of this relationship is described as a "resilience" or "protective" factor.

Mediating factors that are independently capable of producing distress are seen as exerting influence through an "independent causes" relationship. In this second type of mediating relationship, resultant distress is increased in additive fashion, without a significant interaction between etiological and mediating factors.

A "potentiation" relationship represents a third type of interaction possibility, in which a factor interacts with the etiological factor to heighten the PTSD reaction beyond the simple additive effects of the two factors. Thus, the mediating variable acts as both a vulnerability factor and an independent cause in its contribution to PTSD reactivity. Other factors may be influential through an "indirect" route, in which the mediating variable has no direct or interactive effects, but its presence increases the probability of trauma exposure.

The primary purpose of such a formulation is to organize etiological and mediating PTSD factors into an overarching conceptual model to facilitate clinical and research efforts across types of traumatic experiences. To the extent that such a general model of PTSD etiology "fits" the data in the various trauma groups, it is applicable for identifying the relevant foci for assessment and treatment.

Assessment Considerations

Implications from the model can be applied to assessing both ecopathology and psychopathology. In keeping with the interactive emphasis of the model, heterogeneity of trauma experiences is assumed, so that survivors receive clinical assessment appropriate for the uniqueness of their particular trauma exposure. Comprehensive assessment of the chronology and details of the actual trauma(s) is vital. Since the model places critical emphasis upon the nature and intensity of the immediate crisis reaction for determining the likelihood of acute PTSD, thorough assessment of the individual's affective, cognitive, and behavioral responses during the trauma is also essential.

The model further implies that the individual's history of prior trauma exposure is critical for comprehensive assessment. Given the various possible routes for influence by mediating variables, previous traumatization may be a powerful determinant of PTSD reactivity through one or more of them. For example, it may serve indirectly to increase risk for exposure. When a traumatic experience is subsequently encountered, prior trauma history may then also act as a vulnerability or potentiating factor.

Other potential mediating factors in the biological, social, and individual domains also require attention during clinical assessment. For example, evaluating the trauma survivor's family background for history of psychological disorders and significant family dysfunction is important. Family factors, both genetic and social, may be implicated in intergenerational transmission of risk for individual psychopathology. Similarly, levels of social support and intercurrent life events should be assessed, so that current, modifiable sources of potential vulnerability and resilience can be evaluated.

Symptomatic assessment efforts need to include attention to the classic features of traumatic responding: patterns of intrusion, avoidance, and arousal. Although dichotomous assignment of trauma survivors to PTSD-positive and PTSD-negative diagnostic groups is often important for research purposes, this procedure may impose an undesirable element of arbitrariness in some evaluations for clinical purposes. For clinical applications, it may be useful to conceptualize the number and intensity of PTSD symptoms as continuous variables in which considerable variation is to be expected across individuals. In this context, the concept of "partial PTSD" may be useful to describe symptom levels that are clinically relevant but fall short of meeting full diagnostic criteria.

Treatment Considerations

The most obvious implication of our etiological model is that treatment should focus primarily on the nature of the trauma and the survivor's reactions during and after the episode(s). The model implies that the best single predictor of a PTSD reaction is the severity of the traumatic experience. It also posits that trauma needs to be conceptualized as including both "exposure," or objective properties of the event, and uncontrollable immediate personal reactions. The immediate physical and psychological responses thereafter form a conditioned emotional reaction, which is elicited by trauma-related cues.

For many trauma survivors, avoidance of traumatic cues—external cues, as well as physiological or cognitive ones—becomes a guiding principle for maintaining psychological safety. Paradoxically, re-exposure and desensitization to traumatic cues or memories are vital if self-determination is to be regained. Thus, the model implies that traumatic experiences are composed of specific elements that must be processed by the victim, both affectively and cognitively. This sets the stage for using both desensitization and cognitive restructuring in treatment. For chronic cases where avoidant patterns predominate, skills training methods may also be appropriate.

In distinguishing between acute PTSD and chronic forms, the model again allows for the interaction of mediating factors. A prominent issue in this regard is the extent to which the survivor has used extreme coping methods to control PTSD symptoms. For example, using alcohol or other psychoactive drugs to dampen unpleasant levels of anxiety may eventually lead to addiction and its related problems. If interpersonal conflicts are resolved through escape to avoid distressing levels of arousal, ability to function in intimate relationships may become severely impaired.

Comorbid conditions, such as substance abuse, depression, and other anxiety disorders, are to be expected. Unless the comorbid condition has clearly preceded trauma exposure, the implication from the model is that risk for these other disorders is directly linked to PTSD. Accordingly, specific treatment for core PTSD symptoms should be given higher priority in treatment formulation. An exception to this principle may occur when a comorbid condition is blocking efforts at direct treatment of PTSD. Recent history of addictive levels of alcohol or drug use is an example of comorbidity that requires immediate treatment before PTSD treatment can begin.

References

American Psychiatric Association. (1980). *Diagnostic and statistical manual of mental disorders* (3rd ed.). Washington, DC: Author.

American Psychiatric Association. (1987). *Diagnostic and statistical manual of mental disorders* (3rd ed., rev.). Washington, DC: Author.

Astin, M. C., Lawrence, K. Pincus, G., & Foy, D. W. (1990, October). *Moderator variables for PTSD among battered women.* Paper presented at the convention of the International Society for Traumatic Stress Studies, New Orleans.

Blanchard, E. B., Kolb, L., Gerardi, R., Ryan, P., & Pallmeyer, T. (1986). Cardiac response to relevant stimuli as an adjunctive tool for diagnosing post-traumatic stress disorder in Vietnam veterans. *Behavior Therapy, 17,* 592–606.

Breslau, N., Davis, G. C., Andreski, P., & Peterson, E. (1991). Traumatic events and posttraumatic stress disorder in an urban population of young adults. *Archives of General Psychiatry, 48,* 216–222.

Briere, J., & Runtz, M. (1987). Post sexual abuse trauma: Data and implications. *Journal of Interpersonal Violence, 2,* 367–379.

Briere, J., & Zaidi, L. Y. (1989). Sexual abuse histories and sequelae in female psychiatric emergency room patients. *American Journal of Psychiatry, 146,* 1602–1606.

Finkelhor, D., Hotaling, G., Lewis, I., & Smith, C. (1990). Sexual abuse and its relationship to later sexual satisfaction, marital status, religion and attitudes. *Journal of Interpersonal Violence, 4,* 379–399.

Foa, E. B., & Kozak, M. S. (1989). Emotional processing of fear: Exposure to corrective information. *Psychological Bulletin, 99,* 20–35.

Foy, D. W., Osato, S. S., Houskamp, B. M., & Neumann, D. A. (in press). PTSD etiology. In P. A. Saigh (Ed.), *Posttraumatic stress disorder: Behavioral assessment and treatment.* Elmsford, NY: Maxwell Press.

Foy, D. W., Resnick, H. S., Sipprelle, R. C., & Carroll, E. M. (1987). Premilitary, military, and postmilitary factors in the development of combat-related posttraumatic stress disorder. *the Behavior Therapist, 10,* 3–9.

Houskamp, B. M., & Foy, D. W. (1991). The assessment of posttraumatic stress disorder in battered women. *Journal of Interpersonal Violence, 6,* 306–320.

Janoff–Bulman, R. (1985). The aftermath of victimization: Rebuilding shattered assumptions. In C. R. Figley (Ed.), *Trauma and its wake: Vol. 1. The study and treatment of posttraumatic stress disorder* (pp. 15–35). New York: Brunner/Mazel.

Jordan, B. K., Schlenger, W. E., Hough, R., Kulka, R. A., Weiss, D., Fairbank, J. A., & Marmar, C. R. (1991). Lifetime and current prevalence of specific psychiatric disorders among Vietnam veterans and controls. *Archives of General Psychiatry, 48,* 207–215.

Kilpatrick, D. G., & Resnick, H. S. (in press). PTSD associated with exposure to criminal victimization in clinical and community populations. In J. R. T. Davidson & E. B. Foa (Eds.), *PTSD in review: Recent research and future directions.* Washington, DC: American Psychiatric Press.

Kinsey, A. C., Pomeroy, W. B., Martin, C. E. & Gebhard, P. H. (1953). *Sexual behavior in the human female.* Philadelphia: W. B. Saunders.

Kolb, L. C. (1988). A critical survey of hypotheses regarding postraumatic stress disorders in light of recent findings. *Journal of Traumatic Stress, 1,* 291–304.

Koverola, C., Foy, D. W., Heger, A., & Lytle, C. (1990, October). *Relationship of PTSD to sexual abuse trauma assessed by medical findings and child disclosure.* Paper presented at the convention of the International Society for Traumatic Stress Studies, New Orleans.

McLeer, S. V., Deblinger, E., Atkins, M. S., Foa, E. B. & Ralphe, D. L. (1988). Posttraumatic stress disorder in sexually abused children. *Journal of the American Academy of Child and Adolescent Psychiatry, 27,* 650–665.

Robins, L. N. (1990). Steps toward evaluating posttraumatic stress reaction as a psychiatric disorder. *Journal of Applied Social Psychology, 20,* 1674–1677.

Rowan, A. C., Rodriguez, N., Gallers, J., & Foy, D. W. (1990, October). *Sexual abuse exposure factors in the development of PTSD in adult survivors of childhood assault.* Paper presented at the convention of the International Society for Traumatic Stress Studies, New Orleans.

Straus, M. A., & Gelles, R. J. (1986). Societal change and change in family violence from 1975 to 1985 as revealed in two national surveys. *Journal of Marriage and the Family, 48,* 465–479.

2

A Vet Center Experience: Multievent Trauma, Delayed Treatment Type

R. CARL SIPPRELLE

In 1979, when the Van Nuys, California, Vet Center first opened, its counselors were Vietnam veterans who personally understood the anguish of war and had a deep personal commitment to be of service to their fellow survivors. Personnel qualifications were few and guidelines for treatment were even fewer, or so it seemed at the time. An early emphasis on the sociopolitical uniqueness of the Vietnam war contributed to a neglect of the existing literature on trauma from previous wars, violent crime, domestic violence, and natural disasters. Treatment modalities included "peer counseling" and "rap groups," neither clearly specified. Peer counselors were assured that PTSD was eminently treatable and readily responsive to these vague treatment modalities. The failure of other professionals in the private and public sectors to recognize and provide efficacious treatment to Vietnam veterans was attributed to the continuing politics of the war.

Over the next decade, from this beginning, a large and more sophisticated network of treatment centers for Vietnam veterans and their families has evolved. The early model of "peer counseling," "rap groups," and "help without hassles" provided by Vietnam veterans for their peers has been eclipsed by a more professional model, which embraces accountability, research, professionalism, and networking within the mental health community. These changes represent progress at a cost some would call too high.

At this writing, the VA Readjustment Counseling Service operates 197 Vet Centers nationwide, with 818 positions and a fiscal year 1990 budget of 40.6 million. Over 700,000 veterans and family members have been seen since the inception of the program. Although there is variability between centers, a typical center is staffed by a team leader with both administrative and clinical responsibilities, two counselors, an office manager, and adjunct personnel (e.g., volunteers, clinical consultants, and representatives from veteran service organizations and state employment agencies). For a Vet Center of this size, present productivity standards are 31 new Vietnam-era veterans (who may or may not have served "in country"—i.e., within Vietnam) and 264 hours of ongoing assessment and treatment per month. This chapter describes methods used with combat-exposed "in-country" veterans.

Little of the lore that guides practice in Vet Centers has been derived directly through research. It is knowledge that evolved from experience in working with veterans, refined and disseminated by discussions within Vet Center teams and later among Vet Centers at regional training conferences. Since 1979, the Readjustment Counseling Service has published an in-house journal, the *Voice*, to facilitate this communication on a national level. Treatment outcome research with combat-related PTSD has been slow to develop and remains in its infancy. When I was first asked asked to prepare a guide to the assessment and treatment of combat-related PTSD, I balked. I had not made unique research contributions to this literature and doubted that my clinical skills were superior to or distinctive from the skills of my peers. However, I later decided that the guidelines I could describe might be useful to others.

The material presented in this chapter is not a position statement of the VA Readjustment Counseling Service. Universal agreement from my immediate colleagues or other trauma care professionals is not anticipated. It is a guide for those who deal with war-related trauma on a day-to-day basis, in the absence of verified models of assessment and treatment. It may be as naive and simplistic in a few years as our 1979 beliefs and assumptions appear at present.

Combat-Related PTSD

The Vet Center experience has been gained from a specific type of trauma, and this may limit its generalizability to other types of trauma.

Vet Centers serve Vietnam veterans with chronic PTSD, often severe and multiply determined, for whom treatment has been delayed for 10 to 20 years (e.g., Blank, 1982).

Under some circumstances, a single event, such as surviving a violent crime or an environmental disaster, may give rise to symptoms of stress disorder. In Vietnam, during heated periods of the war, riflemen assigned to line infantry companies experienced daily threat of death or injury. In battle, chaos and mayhem prevailed. Many were wounded; many helplessly witnessed the deaths of friends. Unspeakable but unforgettable dramas unfolded. Veterans may have been exposed to the dead and wounded—both combatants and civilians; men, women, and children—many times per week. Many of these casualties were grotesquely mutilated and disfigured by trauma and decay. Following major battles, soldiers loaded the bodies of dead Americans onto pallets; they witnessed the bodies of the enemy being bulldozed into mass graves. Many endured a sustained, unremitting concatenation of this experience for periods up to a year or longer. Their average age at the time was 18.

The secondary trauma of cultural rejection and hostility that confronted men returning from Vietnam may further limit generalizations to other dissimilar trauma experiences. The quality of the post-trauma experience is now known to have a major buffering effect on the development of chronic stress disorder symptoms (Kadushin, 1985).

The perception of a battle-fatigued rifleman, however, is not a sufficient stereotype of the traumatized Vietnam veteran. In the absence of front lines and secure areas, many combat support and service support personnel (e.g., truck drivers, cooks, clerks) were confronted with catastrophic experiences for which they were ill prepared. Although trauma in support personnel was generally more isolated and limited in frequency, it was real, with enduring residual effects.

Intuitively, although one would expect support personnel to be less impaired, they may be symptomatically indistinguishable from their more thoroughly traumatized combatant counterparts. Predisposition may play a differential role in this phenomenon. Perhaps an emotional vulnerability is more operational in the less traumatized support personnel. In contrast, the sustained stress endured by combatants may have been sufficient to overwhelm all exposed (Foy, Resnick, Sipprelle, & Carroll, 1987). Nonetheless, combatants and support personnel share the common experience of secondary trauma following their duty in Vietnam and delayed recognition of their problems.

Unlike natural disasters, with their "act of God" etiology, the trauma endured by combat veterans was man-made—a trauma parameter thought to be associated with more troublesome and persistent emotional residual effects (Figley, 1985). It is true that unlike crime victims and survivors of environmental disasters, veterans were prepared for their experiences through basic training, advanced infantry training, and other more specialized schools. The brutality of Asian counterguerrilla warfare, however, with its ill-defined enemy, the absence of front lines and secure areas, and the apparent lack of purpose and achievable goals, left the training inadequate to the psychological needs of individual soldiers (e.g., Figley & Leventman, 1980). Fulminating, war-related problems went unrecognized and untreated for many years, possibly allowing acute reactions to become chronic in nature.

Assessment

Proper assessment is a critical precursor to effective treatment of combat-related PTSD. A number of disorders have symptoms that overlap with the PTSD symptom cluster and may be easily mistaken for PTSD. A partial list of the disorders that may resemble or co-occur with PTSD include substance abuse disorders, adjustment disorders, anxiety disorders, major depression, and borderline and antisocial personality disorders.

The essential elements of a diagnosis of PTSD are exposure to a stressor that would be expected to generate marked distress in anyone exposed, and the subsequent re-experiencing of the traumatic event in intrusive thoughts, nightmares, or dissociative states. Other DSM-III-R PTSD symptoms, behavior patterns, and dysfunctional lifestyles associated with chronic PTSD are less specific to PTSD. For example, a substance-abusing Vietnam veteran who is alienated from his family of origin and society in general, with a history of multiple failed marriages and vocational instability, poor impulse control, and chronic problems with depression and anger, does not necessarily manifest symptoms of PTSD.

Unfortunately, military histories must be heard with a dash of well-informed skepticism. Individuals may masquerade in the role of traumatized veterans for a number of reasons (e.g., Sparr & Pankratz, 1983; Pary, Tobias, & Lippman, 1987). Some perceive the role as justification for irresponsible or antisocial behavior. Others are seeking compensation for shammed or exaggerated trauma. Still others attempt to assume a distorted, stereotypic role that has been glamorized in the media. It is imperative that a veteran's discharge papers (Form DD-214) be reviewed to establish credibility during assessment. A veteran's failure to produce this document in a reasonable period of time should generate marked skepticism about the alleged military history.

Although the DD-214 will not document specific experiences, it will tend to support or detract from the credibility of an alleged military history and to reveal any gross distortions. Does the DD-214 verify time in Asia? What was the veteran's military occupational specialty (MOS)? What are his personal and unit decorations and specialized schools? Many, if not most, of the case management problems encountered in a Vet Center can be traced to failure to establish credibility with a DD-214 (Melton, 1984).

To make meaningful assessments and initiate useful treatment plans for PTSD, one must be specific about experiences in Vietnam. Among less experienced colleagues, one encounters a "uniformity myth" of Vietnam veterans—a mythical homogeneity of vague and ill-defined experience giving rise to a stereotypic veteran. In reality, veterans encountered a wide range of experiences in Vietnam, and there is no archetypal Vietnam veteran. Listening to inexperienced colleagues, one may hear vague descriptions of traumatized veterans. Upon inquiry, these colleagues are unable to specify the veterans' branch of service, the type of training they had prior to Vietnam, or the primary MOS in which they had been trained. Nor can they describe the actual duty in Vietnam—where in Vietnam these veterans served or with what type of unit. They are unable to describe the social support available to the veterans during and following the war, and are unable to describe with any specificity what allegedly happened in Vietnam to give rise to a chronic stress disorder.

The ability to grasp the essence of a veteran's experience gave the original Vet Center peer counselors an advantage in working with veterans. Their common experience with their clients and familiarity with the order of battle in Vietnam promoted rapport and enhanced their ability to grasp their clients' experience. Therapists who define their role narrowly and technically, and perceive an understanding of these contextual parameters of the war as extraneous to their role, are unlikely to develop and sustain rapport with this population.

The original Vietnam veteran peer counselors readily established and maintained rapport with their clientele. The training of nonveteran counselors for Vet Center positions routinely involves exposure to books and films that enhance the counselors' understanding of the order of battle in Vietnam and the social and political climate in which it occurred. Although a nonveteran therapist is at a disadvantage, such a therapist is capable of working with traumatized veterans, provided that he or she is able to acknowledge this deficit of experience comfortably and nondefensively. To the extent that specific knowledge is required, the therapist must acknowledge the veteran's expertise and allow him to provide the needed information. Although the therapist may lack first-hand experience with war, he or she may still serve as a consultant to a veteran on coping with the residual effects of war in the civilian world. A veteran who balks at a nonveteran therapist typically does so during an initial interview, when the balk is more likely a manifestation of resistance and avoidance than a reaction to the therapist himself or herself.

Experience has shown that nonveteran therapists can work effectively with veterans. Important therapist qualities include a willingness to be exposed to intense anger and agitation, and an ability to dissipate these states in a nonchallenging or nonprovocative manner. An aloof, detached, objective therapeutic stance is usually counterproductive. Effective therapists must be able to skillfully blend the roles of therapist and advocate. Familiarity with the historical context of the Vietnam war and the order of battle in Vietnam are important for Vet Center work, as is familiarity with the issues of ethnic minorities.

Interviews, both structured and nonstructured, have traditionally been the primary diagnostic tool used in the Vet Centers. A sample of a comprehensive structured interview has been presented by Keane, Fairbank, Caddell, Zimering, and Bender (1985). An adaptation of the Structured Clinical Interview for DSM-III-R has also been used extensively in compensation and pension examinations for PTSD (Spitzer & Williams, 1986).

Traditional assessment tools are less often used. The Minnesota Multiphasic Personality Inventory (MMPI; Hathaway & McKinley, 1951) is widely used in VA Medical Center settings and has been included in many PTSD research studies. Although significant findings can be demonstrated for group data (e.g., traumatized veterans can be discriminated from control groups on the basis of MMPI profiles), the utility of the MMPI for making decisions about individual veterans is less impressive (e.g., for compensation purposes, does a given veteran manifest compensable PTSD?) The only other traditional psychological test used with any frequency in the Vet Center has been the Beck Depression Inventory (Beck, Rush, Shaw, & Emery, 1979), which has been used to monitor severity of depression across time, and the Marital Happiness Inventory (Azrin, Naster, & Jones, 1973), which has been used to assess marital satisfaction longitudinally.

PTSD and Other Axis I Disorders

First contact with a Vet Center is often precipitated by stressful current life events, such as marital problems, divorce, loss of job, or death of a significant other. Another common scenario is exacerbation of PTSD symptoms associated with disability or illness in an individual who habitually represses the past by distracting himself with a compulsive whirl of present activity. These life events may be associated with DSM-III-R adjustment disorders if response to the event generates social or industrial impairment or seems disproportionate to the event itself. It is important to be aware of the longitudinal course of PTSD and its potential interaction with current life events.

A chronic and intermittent course is the most common course for combat-related PTSD. After an initial symptomatic period during or immediately following the war, symptoms abate or disappear altogether for weeks, months, or years and then reappear, often unexpectedly. Interviews with older veterans—for example, those who were prisoners of war (POWs) of the Japanese during World War II—demonstrate that this alternating pattern of remission interspersed with symptomatic periods can continue for over 50 years, into the seventh decade of life. Periods of symptom exacerbation may be triggered by specific, combat-related stimuli or by nonspecific stressful life events. The precipitant may be vague, abstract, or unknown, giving the PTSD symptoms a capricious and arbitrary quality that promotes a sense of helplessness. Hence, a typical intake on a new client will reveal not only chronic PTSD but also a co-occurring, precipitating, or exacerbating adjustment disorder.

Substance abuse can amplify and mimic many features of PTSD. Some have suggested that past or present substance abuse co-occurs with combat-related PTSD at rates approaching 100%. Chronic dysphoria, a life characterized by day-to-day endurance, a failure to thrive, inability to maintain intimate relationships, diminished impulse control, and impaired attention and concentration—all features of chronic substance abuse—are often observed in chronic PTSD.

Almost invariably co-occurring with PTSD is depression. The depression may be etiologically unrelated to the PTSD or may represent demoralization associated with the emotional burden of surviving with untreated and chronic PTSD. Frank's (1961) discussion of demoralization is helpful for further consideration of this issue.

Although PTSD may co-occur with disorders of psychotic proportions, few such cases have been observed. Rare cases of co-occurring paranoid schizophrenia, delusional disorder, and bipolar affective disorder are seen. These cases present management problems for which Vet Centers are not adequately staffed and are typically referred to VA Medical Centers. Too few of these individuals have been evaluated and treated to permit any meaningful generalizations to be drawn, other than that they do exist.

PTSD and Axis II Disorders

Personality disorders are widespread among veterans of the Vietnam war. Selective service did not draw randomly from the population of young men during the Vietnam war. Individuals with limited social and educational resources (especially members of ethnic minorities), and progeny of dysfunctional or impoverished families, were over-represented among men drafted to fight the war (Baskir & Strauss, 1981). By virtue of early life trauma and deprivation, many of these men were at risk for manifesting dysfunctional adult behavior, regardless of their military experiences (Van Putten & Yager, 1984). A developmental history characterized by childhood and adolescent trauma, loss, and deprivation should signal a clinician to be alert to the possibility that manifest adult dysfunction is an interactive product of Axis I PTSD and personality disorder.

Without identifiable military trauma and evidence of cognitive re-experiencing of the trauma, the manifest adult dysfunction may be entirely due to early developmental trauma or deprivation. Borderline personality disorder symptoms may so closely resemble PTSD symptoms that there has been some speculation that the two disorders are etiologically related. Perhaps both result from trauma sustained at different developmental periods. The borderline dysfunction may be more generalized and pervasive because of traumatization at an earlier and more vulnerable period, as opposed to the situationally specific, contextually grounded PTSD.

The attraction to weapons and violence, the failure to conform to social norms, the lack of remorse, and diminished sense of empathy to others of the individual manifesting antisocial personality disorder may mimic PTSD. Similarly, the "stable instability"; the impoverished interpersonal support network; the chronic depression and anger, together with episodic outbursts of rage; and the vocational impersistence and failure to establish a mature, adult identity of the individual manifesting borderline personality disorder may mimic PTSD. Also co-occurring with PTSD, although less frequently, are paranoid personality disorder, with symptoms of anger, hypersensitivity, and suspiciousness; narcissistic personality disorder, with symptoms of self-absorption and feelings of entitlement and envy; and schizoid personality disorder, with symptoms of isolation and constriction of affect. The significance of co-occurring Axis II disorders for PTSD treatment planning is discussed below in connection with the integration phase of treatment.

Treatment

Although each veteran is unique, and there is no universal Vet Center treatment plan, a predictable sequence of phases has been noted in the treatment of combat-related PTSD. Individuals present at a Vet Center in a crisis. Although an individual may have experienced stress disorder symptoms for years, these symptoms rarely precipitate entry into treatment. Curiously, many veterans regard these symptoms as "normal."

Typically, treatment is precipitated by an event that is secondary to stress disorder symptoms (e.g., a wife's demand for divorce, termination of employment, or encounters with the criminal justice system associated with violent behavior or alcohol abuse). The first phase of treatment, which co-occurs with assessment, is crisis intervention. Crisis intervention involves stabilizing the crisis and creating, to the extent possible, a secure baseline from which to address the stress disorder symptoms.

The trauma phase follows the crisis intervention phase, and discussion of this phase constitutes the principal focus of this chapter. A final phase, the integration phase, follows the trauma phase and provides the client with an opportunity to adjust to chronic symptoms, explore the impact of trauma on the family, establish and monitor goals, and focus on problem solving and social skills acquisition in a supportive context.

Crisis Intervention Phase

Although there is no fixed formula, most crises can be resolved or stabilized within six weekly sessions. An individual therapy format is used to tailor treatment to the specifics of the crisis. The veteran develops rapport with the therapist in particular and the Vet Center in general. A thorough discussion of crisis intervention is beyond the scope of this chapter and discussion is limited to those aspects relevant to the treatment of chronic PTSD symptoms.

If a veteran's circumstances remain unstable and chaotic (i.e., he moves from one crisis to the next), he should be re-evaluated for undis-

closed substance abuse or character disorder. Some crises preclude further immediate treatment of PTSD. For example, when entry into
treatment is precipitated by an alcohol-related crisis and there is evidence of alcohol dependence, not only must the crisis be resolved, but
the individual must commit himself to an abstinence-oriented recovery
program. As with most psychological disorders, the presence of active
substance abuse renders PTSD relatively untreatable. It remains controversial whether PTSD should be treated during the early weeks and
months of a recovery program. To the extent that the PTSD may have
contributed to the substance abuse, early treatment may facilitate recovery. On the other hand, treatment of PTSD invariably stirs up intense
and powerful affect, which may place an individual at risk for relapse
early in his recovery program.

Suicidal or homicidal ideation may be expressed in the crisis phase
of treatment. Forensic guidelines for protecting the veteran and other
possible victims must be followed. These guidelines require the use of
professional judgment to discriminate authentic threats from manipulat-
ive posturing or symbolic expressions of rage and grief. Therapists must
remember that veterans have survived violent environments, which
have fostered violent ideation and modes of expression. Many, many
threats from veterans are never acted upon. To disallow confidentiality
in response to an impulsive and nonveridical expression of verbal violence may retard or rupture the therapeutic process. Judgment must be
used and is best cultivated by experience and consultation.

Referral for psychiatric services at local VA Medical Centers for
consultation and possible medication or hospitalization may be indicated. The stress of trauma phase work, which may temporarily exacerbate symptoms of agitation, guilt, shame, and despair, should be delayed
in such a case until the veteran is able to resolve acute suicidal or homicidal ideation.

Crises associated with homelessness and unemployment may preclude immediate treatment of PTSD. As Maslow's (1954) hierarchy of
needs suggests, effective treatment of PTSD or any other disorder cannot be accomplished in the context of deprivation of prepotent survival
and safety needs. Before PTSD symptoms can be addressed, family and
community resources need to be mobilized to provide secure shelter and
to ensure that food and other basic requirements can be met on a predictable basis. Similarly, unemployment and its associated uncertainties
seem to preclude effective treatment of PTSD; a successful job search
needs to precede such treatment. The demands of satisfying these needs
prior to trauma phase work are consistent with the ethic of personal responsibility that pervades the trauma phase.

With the resolution of the precipitating crisis, a veteran's motivation to proceed to the second phase of treatment (the trauma phase), may be lost. Although a veteran has the right to terminate treatment with the resolution or stabilization of his crisis, this premature termination is probably associated with the veteran's failure to recognize his stress disorder and its central role in the recurrent crises and general failure to thrive that are characteristic of his postwar life. Alternatively, a veteran may recognize his disorder but be convinced that the disorder is untreatable. Many veterans have had the unsettling experience of stirring up traumatic memories and images in the name of treatment, with no subsequent discernible benefit.

Motivation to continue treatment following the crisis intervention phase is generated by helping the veteran to discover the PTSD-driven themes that have been operating in his civilian life. Rather than seeing the current crisis as an isolated, time-limited event, the veteran is encouraged to see the crisis as the latest enactment of a recurrent PTSD-driven theme. Examples of such themes include problems with authority, poor control of the expression of anger, guilt and self-punishment, or limited capacity for intimacy.

Motivation is also reinforced with a discussion of prognosis and the potential benefits and costs of treatment. A naive promise of full resolution of symptoms is not credible to most veterans, and the therapist will be unable to deliver on such a promise. Combat-related PTSD, 20 years after the trauma is chronic and will continue to color a veteran's life, regardless of treatment. A distinction, however, is drawn between "living well" and "living poorly" with PTSD. Although nightmares and intrusive thoughts may continue, the degree to which they evoke extreme distress can be reduced. The spectrum of PTSD symptoms is discussed, and these symptoms are described as varying in their degree of treatability. For instance, symptoms based on hyperarousal (hypervigilance, sleep disorder, startle response) tend to be very refractory, whereas symptoms based on avoidance and withdrawal (constriction of interest, social withdrawal) respond readily to treatment.

Trauma Phase

War-related PTSD is a complex set of painful and dysfunctional affective and cognitive responses to an extended series of traumatic events. Images and memories of these events and the responses conditioned to them lie unresolved in memory, following a cyclic, self-perpetuating, autonomous agenda of their own that is only intermittently related to the external world (e.g., Green, Wilson, & Lindy, 1985). These memories and the responses conditioned to them may be elicited either by vague and often poorly understood internal stimuli or by external war-related stimuli, such as weapons, Asian people, helicopters, rain, heat and humidity, and objective danger.

Therapy consists of exploration of the traumatic events, the responses conditioned to the events, and the trauma-driven beliefs an individual may have developed about himself, others, and the world. In the process of that emotionally charged exploration, healing may occur through simple desensitization; as a consequence of acquisition of new information; or through cognitive reformulation of events and trauma-driven beliefs about self, others, and the world. Orchestrating an environment in which this can occur is the challenge of therapy.

GROUP THERAPY

Although stress disorder can be treated in either an individual or a group format, the group format has been more successfully used in Vet Centers. The affectively charged process of give and take between a veteran and his peers is seen as the vehicle of healing; hence, the task of the group facilitator is not to interact therapeutically with a veteran, but to engineer an environment in which veterans interact therapeutically with one another. The group facilitator must be able to unobtrusively enter into and withdraw from the content level of the group to influence the process level.

The facilitator accomplishes the task of shaping the group process by a variety of maneuvers, which include providing direct instruction, modeling, and selectively encouraging some types of content and interactions while discouraging others. The therapy, however, is understood to occur in interactions between veterans. When veterans are interacting productively and therapeutically, the group facilitator does not need to do or say anything. Active participation by the facilitator is demanded early in the evolution of a group, when the members are unclear on their roles, or later if a high-quality group begins to lose its focus and therapeutic quality. This general orientation to group therapy is similar to that described by Yalom (1975) in his benchmark work on group therapy.

In the early days of Vet Centers, it was believed that trauma groups should be closed groups of 6 to 10 men who started and completed their trauma group experience together through 2-hour weekly sessions for a specified period of time. Limited therapist resources, client demand, and adjustments to promote flexibility, however, have often resulted in ongoing, open groups into which new members are continually introduced as seasoned members complete their group experience. An unanticipated benefit of this open format has been the opportunity for individuals who have been with the group for a period of time to observe their progress. The mastery they have achieved over their experiences contrasts sharply with the emotional rawness of the trauma of the new members. The open format also allows each client exposure to a larger number of other trauma survivors and their unique circumstances, thus maximizing the opportunity for vicarious learning.

The duration of a trauma group remains controversial. In the absence of relevant research, duration is often determined by available therapist resources and client demand. Duration is also a function of the specific goals of a group. A group focusing exclusively on the trauma phase of therapy may be shorter in duration than a group that sequentially deals with trauma phase issues and follows through into integration phase work. Because extending duration risks dependency, this concern must be carefully monitored.

Early in the evolution of Vet Center trauma groups, the chronicity of war-related trauma was underestimated, and groups were too short in duration. Heated discussions over whether groups should last 8 or 16 weeks characterized that period. Typically, a group contracted for 8 to 16 sessions, and was given the opportunity to contract for further work if the group remained focused and productive at the conclusion of the contractual period. Shorter groups were advocated to reduce problems of dependency. At present, groups are open and long-term. Trauma phase and integration phase issues are blended, with newer members focusing predominantly on trauma phase work and senior members focusing predominantly on integration phase issues.

Although there is no rigid standard, 8 to 16 *months* of weekly meetings are now more typical. Group participants are allowed to decide for themselves when they have achieved maximum group benefits. With healing, competing commitments to other activities and groups become more attractive and compelling; therapy is left behind, much as a child abandons shoes that no longer fit. "Graduates" are encouraged to return as needed for booster sessions or simply to touch base. These visits promote a sense of mastery and provide a model of successful coping for veterans with less time in group.

Group composition has also been controversial. Some have argued for homogeneous groups. Groups limited to men with combat MOSs have been common practice in the Vet Center; as a group, men with combat support and service support MOSs have been perceived as less traumatized and/or as responding to the secondary trauma of cultural rejection rather than combat trauma, and hence they have usually been treated separately. Homogeneity promotes within-group identification and creates a safe environment, in which each man knows that the other participants have had first-hand knowledge of the moral ambiguities and exigencies of war. Combatants suffering moral guilt discuss their experiences only reluctantly with other combatants, and they may not discuss them at all with others, whom they feel are unable to appreciate the circumstances of their actions or lack of action. The price of this homogeneity, however, is that the groups may promote a sense of uniqueness, which reinforces the isolation and estrangement from others that characterize PTSD.

With heterogeneous groups, such as mixtures of traumatized riflemen and less traumatized support personnel, the latter individuals can foster healing in their more impaired coparticipants. They may be less entrenched in bitterness and cynicism, more capable of encouraging and modeling prosocial behavior, more capable of reaching behind their feelings of anger and betrayal, and more capable of responding actively and empathically to the pain of others.

The affective intensity of the groups may have a negative impact on a group facilitator. Facilitators new to trauma may develop a pervasive sense of impending danger and vulnerability, and increased suspicion of the motives of others. McCann and Pearlman (1990) and Figley (1985) have described the acquisition of PTSD-like symptoms by trauma therapists as "vicarious traumatization." This effect can be minimized by having a cotherapist or other colleague with whom to debrief following charged group sessions. The presence of a cotherapist also permits a therapist greater flexibility during group sessions. For example, it becomes possible to attend to personal reactions to group content, or to disengage from the content level and focus on group process.

GROUP DYNAMICS

Early sessions of a group consist of introductions and sharing of military and personal histories. This is typically characterized by enthusiasm and positive affect. Participants often have been so isolated that this may be their first encounter with other Vietnam veterans in many years. Participants are amazed at the similarity of the scripts that appear to be driving their lives. They hear others describe the "secret" symptoms they have attempted to conceal; they see lives characterized by multiple divorces, barren or nonexistent relationships, and frequent job changes due to problems with authority or an inability to tolerate the orderliness and predictability of a conventional life. They share an inability to modulate the expression of anger, a history of drug and alcohol abuse, a generalized mistrust of society and its institutions, suicide attempts, and a general feeling that the last 20 years have been wasted. This phase of interaction and mutual identification, during which group cohesiveness develops, is necessary and preparatory to the work that follows.

Following the introductory period, the group begins its work. There is no one correct way to orchestrate a group. The professional literature contains a number of descriptions of trauma groups for veterans (see, e.g., Scurfield, Corker, Gongla, & Hough, 1984; Jelinek, 1987). Content shifts between war events and current events or premilitary developmental events as a function of participants' interest and the facilitator's clinical orientation. There are, however, common, positive features that occur with high frequency in effective groups.

Effective groups are characterized by veteran-to-veteran interactions rather than veteran-to-facilitator interactions. This is group therapy, not individual therapy with an audience. The group norm is an intense commitment to personal responsibility for problems and their solutions, rather than externalization and blame (e.g., Smith, 1986). Following early sessions, in which discussions of politics and the VA are tolerated to promote group identification and cohesion, these topics are discouraged; they foster a "victim" mentality, with its inherent dynamics of externalization, blame, self–pity, and dependency.

Ineffective groups fail to progress beyond the introductory period described above. Content remains at an emotionally safe level—for example, endless recitation of embellished "drunk-a-logues"; tales of ego-syntonic, violent dyscontrol; angry denouncement of the politics of the war and the antiwar movement; criticism of the VA and the present political leadership; naive fantasies of social justice; and assertions of entitlement. The group develops a collective persona of an angry but powerless victim searching for an external solution to its misery and dysfunction. Ineffective groups are also often (but not always) associated with charismatic, dominant leaders. These groups temporarily satisfy participants, in that they may promote a special and elite identity steeped in entitlement and camaraderie. These groups promote dependency, however, and typically leave participants even more isolated and dysfunctional than they were at baseline.

This dysfunctional group dynamic may be transcended by educating group members about the self-defeating consequences of the victim role they have assumed. Victims are passive objects of external forces, with nonexistent or minimal resources to master or rectify their circumstances. The facilitator may acknowledge that this is a "true" conceptual model of the circumstances of a traumatized veteran, but it is a model with no utility. It is a limiting model that sanctions impairment instead of fostering change and healing. Another, equally valid conceptual model—one with greater utility with respect to healing—is encouraged.

The facilitator encourages group members to substitute the role of survivor for the role of victim. Survivors are seen as traumatized individuals with resources to actively shape their recovery and present circumstances. This conceptual transition from passive, externally determined victim to active, self-determined survivor is difficult for many veterans. Nevertheless, it is important and may to a large extent determine the extent of healing that occurs, both collectively for the group and individually for its participants. Personal responsibility for current circumstances and the tendency to revert to victim behavior must be diligently monitored.

Healing can occur when traumatic events are explored. Because these events are emotionally charged, resistance and avoidance should be anticipated. Although they are usually not necessary, films and videotapes have been used to circumvent persistent resistance and to access war material for the group process. This may be a useful short cut for time-limited groups.

When participants begin to explore traumatic experiences, they commonly experience fears of loss of control. Both therapists and participants need to distinguish carefully between fear of loss of control and real loss of control. The former is almost universal in combatants, the latter less probable. Often a social history will reveal a real loss-of-control problem in late adolescence and early adulthood, often associated with substance abuse. With further maturity and sobriety this very real absence of control abates, leaving many veterans with an unfounded, residual fear of loss of control. If there is a recent history of real loss of control, professional judgment must be exercised regarding the advisability of trauma phase work. Nevertheless, participants correctly intuit that exploration of this material will exacerbate their symptoms. Exploration of trauma may lead to days or weeks of symptom intensification prior to symptom reduction and enhanced functioning.

A central dynamic of war-related PTSD involves anger as a defense against terror, grief, betrayal, and guilt. This may represent counterconditioning, or the substitution of a more desirable response for an undesirable natural response, which began in basic training before veterans ever left the country. It may have continued in Vietnam as combatants learned to numb their terror, grief, betrayal, and guilt with anger and rage. The former states were dysfunctional, in the sense that a surrender to distress in the field jeopardized survival. Twenty or more years later, although the anger has lost its survival value and is socially dysfunctional, it continues with a functional autonomy of its own.

Not only is the anger socially dysfunctional; it may be dysfunctional in the intrapsychic world of the veteran. To the extent that the anger is a defense against a more primary complex of terror, grief, and guilt, it circumvents exposure to this primary stimulus complex, and thus forecloses on the healing processes of desensitization and reformulation. Anger externalizes responsibility for distress, so that external rather than internal problem solutions are implied. Anger undercuts the personal responsibility ethic of the trauma phase. Healing can occur when therapy is able to reach behind the anger and to confront the more primary terror, grief, betrayal, and guilt.

The anger impasse is seductive and difficult for many veterans to grasp, because it contains a compelling emotional truth (e.g., "I and my friends were used terribly in a way that was fundamentally unacceptable. With justification I am bitter and angry"). When veterans are trapped in bitterness and anger, their experiences remain unacceptable; they cycle endlessly between phases of intrusion and denial, which drive chronic PTSD symptoms.

To facilitate movement beyond this surface rage, the facilitator must orchestrate an array of therapeutic processes. Education regarding the defensive function of anger is one element. The relationship between surface anger and the repressed or suppressed feelings of terror, guilt, betrayal, and grief is discussed. Most veterans can recall and describe the onset of this substitution of anger for more vulnerable affective states. This counterconditioning not only was consistent with the traditional role model of male behavior, but was fostered by the military for its tremendous survival value in combat situations.

A major challenge of therapy is to reverse this counterconditioning. Permission giving, modeling, and confrontation are other therapeutic processes that follow the educational prelude. Veterans vary widely in their ability to understand and transcend the anger impasse. This is probably another process variable that determines the degree of both collective healing for the group, and individual healing for its participants.

If a veteran is able to transcend his denial and anger, and to explore his experiences in the empathic presence of his peers, healing may occur. Not only memories were stored, but beliefs about the events and associated beliefs about self, others, and the world. The heat of battle and the turbulence of adolescence provided fertile material for distortions in these beliefs. Although the events were real and immutable, the way in which these events are packaged remains more flexible.

Group content can be emotionally intense. A facilitator must be prepared to witness and assist individuals who experience dramatic and unanticipated symptoms, such as multisensory, dissociative phenomena with overtones of violence and incipient dyscontrol, or acute anxiety or panic states characterized by hyperventilation, severe muscle contractions, and feelings of dyscontrol. Although these states are not inherently dangerous, and actual physical violence in groups is very rare, these overstimulated states are subjectively frightening and are not likely to be intrinsically therapeutic. The veteran feels out of control, and other group members feel helpless. This is a frightening experience in which both the veteran and group members want help getting back in control.

The facilitator may help an overstimulated veteran to recover from these states by calmly communicating that the state is acute and transitory. Verbally and nonverbally, the facilitator communicates control and is not frightened by the symptoms. The facilitator helps the veteran regain control over his symptoms (e.g., "Slow and regulate your breathing") and helps to focus attention away from the internal stimuli that are driving the overstimulated state (e.g., "Open your eyes. . . . Look at me. . . . Would you like a glass of water? . . . Let's stand up and move around"). Parenthetically, the occurrence of these dissociative states is one reason never to allow an intoxicated veteran to remain in a group. Intoxication lowers the threshold for these states, and with the disinhibiting effects of the alcohol, the potential for violence becomes real.

As participants explore their experiences and the influences of these experiences, therapy progresses. Although the specific mechanisms of this healing remain elusive, facilitators' beliefs about these healing mechanisms guide their interactions with the group as they ease into and withdraw from the content level of group interaction.

Interpersonal and group processes such as cohesion, universality, interpersonal learning, and imitative behavior are described by Yalom (1975) as elements of the healing process. Janoff-Bulman (1985) has described healing in terms of cognitive reformulations of beliefs about oneself and the world. Keane et al. (1985) have described a behavioral formulation of PTSD that emphasizes direct therapeutic exposure and an associated model of healing. Complementary processes of sealing over and integration are components of Smith's (1986) discussion of trauma recovery. These explanations are not mutually exclusive, but represent complementary models of complex healing that can be described through many forms of abstraction. An exclusive preoccupation with any single conceptual model may therefore be unnecessarily limiting.

Integration Phase

Chronic, multievent trauma for which treatment was delayed for 10 to 20 years does not respond to a brief course of treatment. Symptom resolution is rarely complete. Earlier in the evolution of my colleagues' and my approach to combat-related PTSD, brief groups lasting 8 to 16 sessions were standard. At the time, these groups appeared effective: Participants talked openly about previously taboo experiences without being overwhelmed with the accompanying affect; guilt abated; intrusive thoughts and nightmares elicited less distress and disruption; and long-term social isolates responded warmly to one another and their families.

Although almost invariably resistant to group termination, most participants complied with termination and left the Vet Center with gratitude for services received. Many if not most of these short-term group participants, however, experienced a relapse of symptoms in a brief period of time. Many, unfortunately, were reluctant to return to the Vet Center. They described a sense of personal failure or a sense of having failed their group and the Vet Center. Gradually, some returned to treatment and helped to expose the naiveté of our initial assumptions regarding the treatment responsiveness of multievent, treatment-delayed trauma.

War-related PTSD may be chronic and symptoms vary in responsiveness to treatment. How can an individual with incompletely treated PTSD be distinguished from an individual who has been comprehensively treated and received maximum benefit? Figley (1985) has argued that one moves from victim to survivor by formulating a "healing theory" that answers five fundamental "victim questions": (1) What happened? (2) Why did it happen? (3) Why did I act as I did then? (4) Why did I act as I have since then? and (5) How will I act if it happens again? A simpler standard has evolved at the Vet Center: If a veteran is able to describe what happened without becoming overwhelmed with grief or rage, and experiences no subjective need for further work, therapy is complete. This does not preclude appropriate affective modulation of his tale. It only means that the modulation is not subjectively overwhelming.

At this writing, treatment has been extended by the addition of the integration phase. This work has been done both in a group format continuing from the trauma phase and in adjunctive individual and family therapy modes. Within the integration phase, trauma work may continue intermittently as previously undigested experiences intrude into consciousness, but the primary focus is on present life. Common themes of the integration phase include the impact of past trauma on the family; goal setting and monitoring; and adjustment to chronic, treatment-refractory symptoms. Support, problem solving, and social skills training form a matrix for these themes. These themes are elaborated individually here, although in a group they form a blend of interwoven themes, with each participant dealing with material appropriate to his circumstances.

As trauma is mastered and recedes into the past, the interpersonal deficits associated with 20 years of social withdrawal and avoidance may inhibit progress on rehabilitation goals and diminish life satisfaction. Problem-solving skills may be poorly developed because of prolonged overreliance on dysfunctional, short-term solutions to life's quandaries, such as aggression and violence, avoidance and flight, and substance abuse. An ongoing group provides an ideal microcosm in which to develop social and problem-solving skills.

Anger and aggressiveness are prominent interpersonal excesses in many veterans. These qualities promoted survival in Vietnam and may even have some effectiveness as short-sighted solutions to civilian problems. Eventually, however, overreliance on aggression alienates employers, colleagues, family, and friends. With feedback from group members, more situationally appropriate assertiveness can be developed and practiced in ongoing groups. As members become more verbal and articulate, they may develop the capacity to bind and express hostile impulses with language rather than acting them out physically.

Benumbed by trauma, many veterans are deficit in their ability to give or receive nurturance; they lack important listening and empathic responding skills. As the group develops trust and cohesiveness, affective bonds develop between members, and they begin to recognize and share their common experiences during and following the war. Awkwardly, they learn to respond to the pain of their fellow veterans. They begin to develop tolerance and patience as they witness one another's struggle. They begin to arrive early for group to socialize in the Vet Center lobby, and they linger in the parking lot after group. Spontaneously, phone numbers are exchanged, and participants begin to meet away from the Center.

Experiences in Asia sensitized many veterans to existential issues at an early age. In isolation, they have puzzled over issues of death, freedom, isolation, and meaninglessness for years (e.g., Yalom, 1980). For some, life intermittently dominated by moment-to-moment survival in a free-fire zone was simple, intense, and intoxicating. The urgent intensity of war and the intimate relationships it bred underlie the apparent contradictions of veterans who suffer the memories of war while simultaneously longing to return. The group can serve as a forum to explore these issues.

TRAUMA AND THE FAMILY

In recent years, the chronicity and treatment-refractory quality of multi-event, treatment-delayed trauma have led to an interest in veterans' families. Are there contextual parameters within veterans' families that influence the course of stress disorder symptoms? What is the impact of trauma on nontraumatized family members? What role do family members play in recovery from or perpetuation of symptoms in traumatized veterans? This work is typically done with a veteran and his family in a family therapy format, rather than as part of an integration phase group. Couples groups are a recent innovation, but at present our experience with such groups is minimal, and no conclusions or generalizations are offered here.

A malignant contagion from trauma survivors to others intimately involved in their lives is now widely recognized (e.g., Figley, 1985). Many symptoms in the PTSD spectrum are interpersonal in nature, such as constriction of interest, feelings of detachment, restricted affect, and irritability. These symptoms have a direct impact on family relationships. Similarly, veterans' hypervigilance and exaggerated sense of danger have a powerful shaping effect on their families' beliefs about personal vulnerability in a capricious and dangerous world. The secondary substance abuse to which so many veterans have succumbed also shapes family patterns of behavior in characteristic ways. The high rates of divorce and domestic violence hint at the corrosive effects of trauma on families (Matsakis, 1989).

Some research supports the idea that family systems may have a powerful effect on the manifestation of PTSD symptoms (e.g., Williams & Williams, 1987). Traumatized veterans cannot exist independently of the systems in which they live. Dysfunctional men are at risk for forming relationships with dysfunctional women. Ultimately, these couples become entangled in habitual negative patterns of interaction.

One dynamic is rooted in the exaggerated sense of danger that distorts many veterans' perceptions of the world. In a dangerous and unpredictable world, constant vigilance and a readiness to react decisively are demanded. Women and children are perceived as naive and trusting; thus, the veteran may see his role as that of protector. His competence is defined and amplified by the incompetence of his family. He leads, they follow. Family patterns and activities are geared to his needs; women and children are secondary satellites in his orbit. If this formulation of family life is challenged or rejected by family members, danger is heightened, vigilance is intensified, and the veteran escalates his struggle for control.

Another common dynamic revolves around withdrawal and restricted capacity to give and receive nurturance. A veteran's oblique expression of love (e.g., in the roles of protector and provider) may fail to satisfy the emotional needs of his family. Their more emotional expression of love and need are unsettling to him; their intimacy may provoke feelings of danger and vulnerability, and thus may stimulate further withdrawal. If the system is challenged by family members—for example, if family members should detach themselves from the dysfunctional system and attempt to meet their needs independently of the veteran—danger escalates; the veteran feels out of control and often effectively engineers intensified isolation of his family from others.

GOAL SETTING AND MONITORING

As stated above, the sense of having "wasted" the last 20 years is common in Vet Center clients. Few have established enduring relationships or satisfying careers. Many look back on a lengthy series of painful failures. An acquired sense of helplessness and futility is common. As veterans achieve a mastery over traumatic experiences, they often need rehabilitation to maximize the potential that is revealed.

With healing, veterans become more receptive to VA benefits for which they are been qualified but that they have been unwilling to pursue or accept. Many request and are granted compensation for social and industrial impairment associated with PTSD; and/or vocational rehabilitation benefits enabling further education or training. To the extent that obtaining these benefits requires patience and persistence, support and encouragement are provided. Establishing and monitoring progress toward both short- and long-term goals help to break the inertia of the last 20 years and to diminish helplessness and futility. When this is done in a group setting, the approval of peers can motivate and energize the process.

With refractory veterans deeply mired in helplessness, a careful distinction must be made between depression and self-pity. A cognitive model focusing on beliefs about self, others, and the future is useful. With depression, which is characterized by negative beliefs about self, others, and the future, a nurturant stance may be useful while the depression is addressed. With self-pity, which is characterized by positive beliefs about self and negative beliefs about others and the world, a nurturant stance is contraindicated; in this case, confrontation is demanded. As group members begin to recognize self-pity in themselves and others, they appear to enjoy the confrontations that ensue.

Confrontation is essential for a small but significant proportion of Vet Center clients who can drain the resources of a Center. These men are minimally traumatized service or combat support personnel who claim to suffer from severe PTSD symptoms but are unable to credibly describe significant personal trauma that would justify these symptoms. PTSD-related impairment, if present, is dwarfed by Axis II character pathology. They are deeply mired in an angry, self-pitying, victim complex. Their agenda is not to transcend their Vietnam experience and place it appropriately in the past but to amplify and embrace it, making a career out of the identity of "traumatized veteran."

These men typically come from dysfunctional families of origin. This is a borderline struggle to erect and maintain an identity that has been glamorized in recent years and that some feel mitigates responsibility for antisocial or inappropriate behavior. To the extent that such a veteran is a viable treatment case at all—that is, to the extent that the veteran and therapist can agree on realistic and achievable treatment goals—an approach characterized by constant goal setting and monitoring and by ongoing, unremitting confrontation of the self-pitying, victim attitude is required (Merback, 1984). These men may respond to a nurturant and nondemanding therapy relationship with increased dependency and entitlement, as well as an escalation of acting-out behavior. Marked Axis II character problems lower the treatability and prognosis for true trauma residuals.

CHRONIC SYMPTOMS

The emphasis of therapy in the trauma phase is on what happened in the past; it explores traumatic events and their contextual parameters. In contrast, the integration phase is present-focused; the emphasis here is on how to live with past trauma through symptom management.

Symptoms associated with hyperarousal tend to be refractory. These symptoms include sleep disorder, hypervigilance, and exaggerated startle response. With severe sleep disorder, other symptoms are exacerbated, such as irritability and impairment of concentration. Some have suggested focal behavioral interventions for these symptoms (e.g.,

Perconte, 1988), but symptom reduction from these procedures is often transient. Psychiatric medications can suppress these hyperarousal symptoms to some degree, but there are frequently problems with side effects, dependency, and tolerance. Furthermore, because most veterans are substance abusers or are in recovery from substance abuse, medications must be used judiciously.

Recurrence of memories in the form of intrusive thoughts and nightmares typically continues, albeit at a reduced frequency. These memories also come to be described as less distressing and disruptive. For example, prior to treatment, a veteran may describe awakening from nightmares in a state of terror that dissipates only slowly over the course of the following day. He is unable to return to sleep, and the following day is raw with irritability, apprehensiveness, and fatigue. Following treatment, he may describe awakening in a state of terror but quickly being able to orient and calm himself; he returns to sleep with no residuals extending into the following day.

Guilt may remain following an extended course of treatment. As the distortions attributed to events are corrected, however, and unrealistic and inflexible standards of conduct are explored with peers, the excruciating moral guilt that previously drove self-defeating and self-destructive behavior assumes more tolerable and situationally appropriate proportions.

The emphasis is not on achieving a symptom-free state, but on "living well" with residual symptoms. Participants learn that intensification of symptoms is a signal to attend to and respond to accumulating stress. For combat veterans, PTSD symptoms often have become a final common pathway for the expression of stress in any domain of life. Conflict with spouses, children, or employers; financial problems, excessive demands on the job; illness; and inadequate rest and recreation may all be expressed through intensification of PTSD symptoms. In the integration phase, the participant with chronic PTSD learns that his tolerance for stress has been compromised. Intensification of symptoms becomes a signal to monitor one's circumstances closely. Participants are encouraged to co-opt the Alcoholics Anonymous slogan "Keep it simple." Problems are aggressively confronted as they arise and are not allowed to accumulate.

To "live well" with multievent, treatment-delayed trauma is a difficult but achievable goal. Fifty years after surviving the Bataan death march and a subsequent 42-month internment at slave labor in Japanese POW camps, a 70-year-old veteran was interviewed. He stated that he would not repeat his experiences for a million dollars, but recalled them as the most enriching, ennobling experiences of his entire life.

Acknowledgments

The ideas described herein evolved from experience with over 4,000 Vietnam veterans in a southern California Vet Center sequentially located in Van Nuys (1980–1981), Northridge (1981–1987), and Sepulveda (1987–present). Presently, it is one of two Vet Centers in the nation located on VA Medical Center grounds. The ideas were distilled from discussions with past and present Vet Center employees, including David Alcaras, Francisco Cortinas, David Culmer, Rodney Dalton, Robert Duncan, Roger Melton, Alison Passalaqua, and Mark Waind.

References

Azrin, N. H., Naster, B. J., & Jones. R. (1973). Reciprocity counseling: A rapid learning-based procedure for marital counseling. *Behaviour Research and Therapy, 11,* 365–382.

Baskir, L. M., & Strauss, W. A. (1981). The Vietnam generation. In A. D. Horne (Ed.), *The wounded generation: America after Vietnam* (pp. 5–15). Englewood Cliffs, NJ: Prentice-Hall.

Beck, A. T., Rush, A. J., Shaw, B., & Emery, G. (1979). *Cognitive therapy of depression.* New York: Guilford Press.

Blank, A. S. (1982). Apocalypse terminable and interminable: Operation Outreach for Vietnam veterans. *Hospital and Community Psychiatry, 33,* 913–918.

Figley, C. R. (1985). From victim to survivor: Social responsibility in the wake of catastrophe. In C. R. Figley (Ed.), *Trauma and its wake: Vol. 1. The study and treatment of posttraumatic stress disorder* (pp. 398–415). New York: Brunner/Mazel.

Figley, C. R., & Leventman, S. (1980). *Strangers at home: Vietnam veterans since the war.* New York: Praeger.

Foy, D. W., Resnick, H. S., Sipprelle, R. C., & Carroll, E. M. (1987). Premilitary, military, and postmilitary factors in the development of combat-related posttraumatic stress disorder. *the Behavior Therapist, 10,* 3–9.

Frank, J. (1961). *Persuasion and healing.* Baltimore: Johns Hopkins University Press.

Green, B. L., Wilson, J. P., & Lindy, J. D. (1985). Conceptualizing posttraumatic stress disorder: A psychosocial framework. In C. R. Figley (Ed.), *Trauma and its wake: Vol. 1. The study and treatment of posttraumatic stress disorder* (pp. 53–72). New York: Brunner/Mazel.

Hathaway, S. R., & McKinley, J. C. (1951). *MMPI manual* (rev. ed.). New York: Psychological Corp.

Janoff-Bulman, R. (1985).The aftermath of victimization: Rebuilding shattered assumptions. In C. R. Figley (Ed.), *Trauma and its wake: Vol. 1. The study and treatment of posttraumatic stress disorder* (pp. 15–35). New York: Brunner/Mazel.

Jelinek, J. M. (1987). Group therapy with Vietnam veterans and other trauma victims. In T. Williams (Ed.), *Posttraumatic stress disordes: A handbook for clinicians* (pp. 209–221). Cincinnati: Disabled American Veterans.

Kadushin, C. (1985). Social networks, helping networks, and Vietnam veterans. In S. M. Sonnenberg, A. S. Blank, & J. A. Talbot (Eds.), *The trauma of war: Stress and recovery in Vietnam veterans.* New York: American Psychiatric Press.

Keane, T. M., Fairbank, J. A., Caddell, J. M., Zimering, R. T., & Bender, M. E. (1985). A behavioral approach to treating posttraumatic stress disorder in Vietnam veterans. In C. R. Figley (Ed.), *Trauma and its wake: Vol. 1. The study and treatment of posttraumatic stress disorder* (pp. 257–294). New York: Brunner/Mazel.

Maslow, A. H. (1954). *Motivation and personality.* New York: Harper.

Matsakis, A. (1989). Surveying the damage: The effects of PTSD on family life. *VA Practitioner, 6,* 75–81.

McCann, I. L., & Pearlman, L. A. (1990). Vicarious traumatization: A framework for understanding the psychological effects of working with victims. *Journal of Traumatic Stress, 3,* 131–149.

Melton, R. (1984). Differential diagnosis: A common sense guide to psychological assessment. Part I: Factitious posttraumatic stress disorder. *Voice, 5,* 1–4.

Merback, K. (1984). A Vet Center dilemma: Posttraumatic stress disorder and personality disorders. *Voice, 5,* 6–7.

Pary, R., Tobias, C., & Lippman, S. (1987). Recognizing shammed and genuine posttraumatic stress disorder. *VA Practitioner. 4,* 37–43.

Perconte, S. T. (1988). Stages of treatment in PTSD. *VA Practitioner. 5,* 47–57.

Scurfield, R. M., Corker, T. M., Gongla, P. A., & Hough, R. L. (1984). Three post-Vietnam "rap/therapy" groups: An analysis. *Group, 8,* 3–21.

Smith, J. R. (1986). Sealing over and integration: Modes of resolution in the post–traumatic stress recovery process. In C.R. Figley (Ed.) *Trauma and its wake: Vol. 2. Traumatic stress theory, research, and intervention* (pp. 20–38). New York: Brunner/Mazel.

Sparr, L., & Pankratz, L. D. (1983). Factitious posttraumatic stress disorder. *American Journal of Psychiatry, 140,* 1016–1019.

Spitzer, R. L., & Williams, J. B. W. (1986). *Structured Clinical Interview for DSM-III-R: Post-traumatic stress disorders.* New York: New York State Psychiatric Institute.

Van Putten, T., & Yager, J. (1984). Posttraumatic stress disorder: Emerging from the rhetoric. *Archives of General Psychiatry, 41,* 411–413.

Williams, C. M., & Williams, T. (1987). Family therapy for Vietnam veterans. In T. Williams (Ed.), *Posttraumatic stress disorder: A handbook for clinicians* (pp. 221–233). Cincinnati: Disabled American Veterans.

Yalom, I. D. (1975). *The theory and practice of group psychotherapy* (2nd ed.). New York: Basic Books.

Yalom, I. D. (1980). *Existential psychotherapy.* New York: Basic Books.

3

Assessment and Treatment of Combat-Related Post-Traumatic Stress Disorder in a Medical Center Setting

EDWARD M. CARROLL and DAVID W. FOY

It is the purpose of this chapter to describe the management and treatment of PTSD in a medical center setting. In particular, we focus on treatment issues and strategies that are germane to an inpatient setting. The discussion is primarily based on our experience treating combat-related PTSD within a VA Medical Center. However, much of the material is equally relevant to other PTSD populations and inpatient settings. The first sections of the chapter concern preliminary treatment considerations, such as the physical and social context of client management, critical client and expectancy variables, and important therapist characteristics that can affect treatment. Later sections describe specific assessment and intervention techniques, as well as ways to promote treatment generalization following discharge.

Inpatient Treatment Setting

Physical Setting

The physical environment of a medical center setting usually consists of a variety of inpatient wards. The inpatient units vary in terms of their specialization and the types of physical and psychological problems they address. Psychiatric inpatient units may specialize in the treatment of certain types of psychological disorders (e.g., substance abuse, affective disorders), or they may be general wards that treat all psychiatric admissions to the medical center. A notable example of a successful inpatient unit specializing in the treatment of PTSD is the Menlo Park (California) Vietnam Veterans Treatment Program, which has been in continuous operation for over 10 years (Berman, Price, & Gusman, 1982). This program now serves as a prototype for the development of new PTSD treatment units in other medical centers. Although a number of other VA Medical Centers now provide inpatient wards that specialize in the treatment of PTSD, the majority of patients with combat-related problems are initially hospitalized on more generalized wards. Referral to a specialized PTSD unit usually occurs later in treatment.

Patient Population

The patient population on general psychiatric units is characterized by a wide variety of psychopathology. Patients with severe thought disorders (e.g., schizophrenia, organic brain syndromes) are common, as are patients with disabling affective disorders. Increasingly, persons with extreme types of character pathology are residents of VA inpatient wards.

In terms of the clinical management of patients with PTSD, it is important to assess and address their feelings about being on an inpatient unit shortly after admission. This is especially critical with PTSD patients who are entering the medical center for the first time. The observation of other patients with "very crazy" behavior can alarm PTSD patients and trigger feelings that they do not belong in the setting. Denial and treatment avoidance are often long-standing complications to the successful treatment of PTSD. Exposure to other patients with severe psychopathology can provide avoidant PTSD patients with an easy excuse for leaving the treatment setting. Thus, it is important to be aware of each patient's potential reaction to the inpatient social environment and to make it an initial focus of the treatment plan, in order to prevent premature elopement from treatment. Reassurance and support of the PTSD patient's decision to pursue intensive treatment may need to be provided repeatedly during the first week of hospitalization. An effort to educate PTSD patients about the benefits of inpatient treatment and to assist differentiation of their clinical needs from those of other inpatients will help reduce the risk of elopement from the medical center setting.

Treatment Team

The composition of the treatment team is another aspect of the setting that is critical to the outcome of PTSD therapy. Most often, the treatment team is multidisciplinary, including psychiatrists, psychologists, social workers, nurses, and aides or technicians. Psychiatrists are usually responsible for formulating the medication regimen aimed at reducing patients' symptoms and for monitoring patients' physical health. Psychologists most often perform psychological assessments to assist in diagnosis and treatment planning, and they contribute to the treatment plan by formulating behavioral and psychosocial interventions. Social workers provide assessments of social and environmental resources and help develop provisions for housing, income, and family support. Nursing service is responsible for continuous patient care and monitoring of patients' behavior. The members of all services may provide psychotherapy and individual supportive therapy according to their training and experience.

There are several advantages to working in an inpatient setting. The multidisciplinary team element ensures that each patient has direct access to a variety of mental health care providers and can be monitored 24 hours a day in times of crisis. The fact that the patient is assessed from a variety of mental health perspectives makes the treatment plan multifaceted; in other words, there are a number of professionals who know the patient and can provide ready consultation in regard to treatment planning. The combination of medication, psychological intervention, and the development of social supports can be more readily provided by an interdisciplinary treatment team than by an individual outpatient practitioner. Although consultations from other services may be available to the outpatient clinician, they are not provided by colleagues who necessarily have personal knowledge of the patient. In addition, the 24-hour monitoring of patient behavior allows for ongoing evaluation of interventions' effectiveness and is a tremendous help in managing patient crises. For example, nightmares and sleep problems are defining characteristics of PTSD. The observations of the nursing staff on the night shift can greatly assist the effort to evaluate treatment efficacy. Although self-report and feedback from significant others may assist an outpatient clinician's assessment of intervention effectiveness, the daily nursing report is more immediate and less susceptible to bias.

Crisis management also is enhanced in an inpatient setting. The initiation of PTSD treatment (e.g., flooding procedures) is often accompanied by a significant increase in subjective distress and suicidal ideation. It is a comfort to both patients and clinicians to know that external controls are available 24 hours a day to protect the patients against impulsive behavior. It may become necessary during the treatment of some severe cases to work out a 24-hour monitoring system with other staff members. This can help remove the temptation to commit self-destructive acts and provide supportive counseling on an "as-needed" basis. In turn, this allows patients to continue in therapy further than they might be able to do in the absence of therapeutic team support. Rather than leaving treatment because of the significant initial distress of therapy, patients can learn to tolerate traumatic memories and to lead life under less stressful conditions.

Although there are clear advantages to a multidisciplinary treatment setting, there are also potential drawbacks. Perhaps the most critical of these is the manner in which interpersonal dynamics and conflicts between staff members can negatively influence patient care. It would be ideal if all members of the various disciplines cooperated uniformly in team management of patient care. In the real world, however, "turf" battles and personal dislikes can affect the decision making and functioning of the treatment team.

A frequent area of interdisciplinary conflict in the treatment of PTSD patients is the use of medications. It is not surprising that a treating psychiatrist will often utilize antidepressant and tranquilizing medications when faced with a patient who reports high levels of subjective distress. However, other mental health clinicians may view the use of pharmacotherapy as short-sighted and as interfering with the behavioral treatment objective of extinguishing anxiety reactions to trauma-related stimuli. The more immediate effects of sedating medications can make the longer process of psychotherapy an unwelcome approach in the eyes of many staff members. The short-term gains, however, need to be balanced with the long-term risk of medication side-effects. Also, there is the potential for a chronic reliance upon medications and an avoidance of the painful process of working through the emotional sequelae of traumatic experiences. This is not to say that medications cannot be useful when balanced with behavioral interventions and consideration of the patient's clinical condition (cf. Friedman, 1991; Rosen & Bohon, 1990). Patients with PTSD can vary considerably in terms of their responsiveness to and need for medication, group therapy, individual therapy, and social supports. The ability of the treatment team members to cooperate in their treatment efforts is essential to a positive outcome. If the climate of the treatment team is conflictual and dominated by interdisciplinary competition, intervention efforts will be severely compromised.

The support and cooperation of the nursing service are also critical factors in the quality of care provided to PTSD patients. The early phases of behavioral treatment frequently result in intensified distress. Sudden increases in suicidal and homicidal feelings are not uncommon. Obviously, this places an added burden upon staff members who cover the unit for 24 hours. There is no substitute for discussing these possibilities prior to the start of behavioral treatment. As many staff members as possible should receive an explanation of the treatment process and be informed about the possibility of periodic crises. There is always the chance that some members of staff will view an intervention negatively and will not be favorable toward incurring increased risk for crisis. However, it is likely that the majority of the staff will provide coverage and support if the treatment plan is thoroughly explained and cooperation is solicited. It is recommended that prior to treatment, careful consideration be given to staff members' attitudes toward the intervention, so that those who are most interested and motivated can be assigned to cover the PTSD patient. If uninterested or hostile staff members are assigned, then increased risk of treatment sabotage is to be expected.

Patient Variables

The treatment of PTSD patients in an inpatient setting is influenced by several important patient variables, including: (1) comorbidity, or the presentation of multiple clinical syndromes; (2) factors related to compensation seeking; and (3) patient expectancies. In contrast to outpatient settings, inpatient units tend to receive patients exhibiting more severe forms of psychopathology. In addition to greater severity of symptoms, frequently there are problems in determining a clear diagnosis. Although some patients will be admitted with clear-cut PTSD problems, the majority present with multiple clinical problems, only some of which may be combat-related sequelae. Differential diagnosis and the determination of clinical severity are critical components of treatment planning.

Comorbidity Considerations

Given the chronic nature of combat-related PTSD, it is not sufficient to focus the psychological evaluation only on the question of whether or not the patient exhibits symptoms of PTSD. It is necessary to identify the full range of clinically significant problems. The diagnostic categories used by prior clinicians should be reviewed thoroughly and should not be accepted without question. Misdiagnosis of PTSD was and still is common, especially in evaluations conducted prior to 1980, when diagnoses of schizophrenia or personality disorder were often used for PTSD cases. On the other hand, records showing the single diagnosis of PTSD should not blind the assessor to the potential for concomitant problems, such as substance abuse or personality disorders. Major depressive episodes and other types of anxiety disorders can frequently be identified when conducting a thorough diagnostic assessment of patients with potential PTSD. In an inpatient setting, comorbidity is the rule rather than the exception.

Personality disorders often become relevant to the differential diagnosis of combat-related PTSD. Long-standing characterological deficits may be diagnostic alternatives to PTSD or may coexist and interact with PTSD. Antisocial and borderline traits, in particular, are common considerations when evaluating Vietnam veterans. Crucial to the determination of the relevance of personality factors is the nature of the particular patient's premilitary functioning. Signs of personality disorder usually emerge during childhood or adolescent developmental periods. It is extremely useful to obtain a developmental history from a variety of sources, including the patient and relatives or friends who are familiar with the patient's behavior prior to military service. Indications of developmental instability, pronounced family conflict, early substance abuse, repeated trouble with authority, school problems, and psychological help seeking should alert the assessor to the potential role of characterological problems in the patient's current clinical picture. Axis II personality disorder diagnoses should only be made when there is solid historical evidence of developmental problems. Current behavioral indicators of personality disorder may be related to military service rather than premilitary adjustment. For example, many Vietnam combat veterans with "healthy" premilitary functioning will evidence social alienation, violent outbursts, substance abuse, distrust of authority, and dysfunctional social adjustment. Obtaining a good developmental history will facilitate determination of whether these problems are related to military experiences or are lifelong patterns of behavior.

Substance abuse problems have become ubiquitous as confounding factors in the treatment of most mental health disorders, and the treatment of PTSD is no exception. In many cases, substance abuse will be found to be a secondary problem to PTSD. Some veterans may use street drugs and alcohol as a way of self-medicating psychological distress. In other cases, substance abuse may be found to be a primary problem that may coexist with PTSD. Once again, a detailed examination of each patient's history will facilitate differential diagnosis.

It is not uncommon to find cases of PTSD misdiagnosed as schizophrenia or some other type of thought disorder. The presence or absence of legitimate hallucinations, delusions, or formal thought disorder is pivotal in distinguishing PTSD from psychotic disorders. Severe cases of PTSD may include dramatic re-experiencing of traumatic events (e.g., flashbacks), which can be misinterpreted as hallucinations. Examining the content of these experiences as to whether or not they are trauma-related can help establish the differential diagnosis.

Since relatively few patients evidence co-existing problems of PTSD and schizophrenia, the frequency and nature of such cases have received scant empirical attention. However, this population deserves more research attention. Vulnerability for the onset of schizophrenia occurs in the early 20s; of course, this is the age at which many Vietnam veterans performed their military service. It is reasonable to hypothesize that a subset of veterans experienced their first psychotic episode in Vietnam and that the content of their thought disorder is combat-related. Although rare in occurrence, this particular dual diagnosis may be particularly important to treatment planning. Current experience suggests that even when such patients have been responsive to antipsychotic medications, specific behavioral treatment for PTSD symptoms increases risk for relapse and regression. In these cases, patients may not be able to tolerate even initial attempts to process trauma-related clinical material.

Treatment Considerations for Patients with Dual Diagnoses

The following recommendations are intended as general guidelines for directing the treatment of patients with PTSD and concurrent clinical syndromes.

PTSD AND SUBSTANCE ABUSE

Substance abuse problems will need to be addressed prior to PTSD treatment in most instances. Whether substance abuse is primary (i.e., an independent and/or pre-existing problem) or secondary (i.e., a form of self-medication of PTSD distress) in nature, patients need to be substance-free during the period of active PTSD intervention. It is probably unrealistic and overexclusionary to demand lengthy pretreatment sobriety. However, a patient should be thoroughly detoxified and free from illicit substance use for several weeks prior to PTSD treatment. Inpatient treatment has some advantage over outpatient treatment in this regard. The inpatient treatment modality allows for closer monitoring of the patient's daily behavior and gives a clinician relatively more control over the patient's environment. Thus, an inpatient setting may be recommended for those PTSD patients with severe or chronic substance abuse problems.

PTSD AND CHARACTER PATHOLOGY

Patients who also exhibit Axis II psychopathology present especially difficult clinical management problems. There is no reason, however, to delay PTSD treatment efforts because of characterological symptoms. Problems with treatment resistance, hostility, threatened violence, and staff conflict will demand staff attention and a coordinated system of patient management, but such problems do not necessitate delay of treatment. To the contrary, efforts to sabotage treatment should be expected from patients with personality disorders. It is often critical to persevere with treatment efforts while managing problematic acting-out behavior. Delaying or stopping treatment may negatively reinforce the dysfunctional behavior and make future treatment efforts even more difficult.

PTSD AND PSYCHOSIS

If the patient's initial evaluation indicates severe forms of thought disorder in addition to symptoms of PTSD, the prognosis for successful treatment of PTSD, unfortunately, is poor in our experience. Even when medications effectively reduce the severity of thought disorder, subsequent efforts to treat the PTSD problems usually result in regression and an exacerbation of psychotic symptoms. Because there may be exceptions, it is recommended that this type of dual-diagnosis patient be treated first with antipsychotic medications and that the treatment of PTSD be attempted only after several weeks of stabilization. However, PTSD treatment efforts should be discontinued if psychotic symptoms start to return. It may be that patients with severe forms of thought disorder cannot tolerate the added stress of confronting traumatic experiences.

PTSD AND AFFECTIVE DISORDER

The combination of PTSD and affective disorder is a very frequent type of dual diagnosis in an inpatient setting. Most often, the patient will be started on antidepressant medications prior to PTSD treatment efforts. Subsequently, behavioral and medication interventions may be used concurrently with beneficial effects. If PTSD treatment efforts prove successful in reducing trauma-related distress and increasing coping behaviors, the medications may be tapered off on a trial basis in order to assess whether they are still independently useful. This is best achieved while the patient remains in an inpatient setting, where symptom monitoring can take place on a 24-hour basis. If the medication reduction process proves problematic, outpatient follow-up and rehabilitation planning can proceed in conjunction with continued medication consultation.

Compensation–Pension Considerations

The possibilities of malingering and of secondary gain factors have become increasingly prominent in the management of PTSD cases. Hospital benefits and financial compensation can be obtained from the VA for some cases of combat-related PTSD. Although there are many deserving veterans who rightfully obtain compensation, there are a troublesome few who attempt to misuse the system. In recent years, considerable media attention has been paid to the problems of Vietnam veterans. Part of this media attention has included detailed descriptions of PTSD; as a result, it has become possible to fake or exaggerate trauma-related symptoms. Several studies have shown that many veterans can falsely present these symptoms in a manner that is difficult to detect, even by experienced clinicians.

The problem of malingering does not apply only to combat-related PTSD assessment. The psychological sequelae of all types of trauma (e.g., rape, airline disaster, etc.) can be financially compensated by litigation; they have become a highly recognized and utilized part of litigation. Again, there are many who deserve financial compensation, but there are others who exploit the growing awareness of trauma-related psychological problems.

Prior to initiating treatment procedures with a PTSD patient, it is well worth the time to carefully examine the patient's motivation for inpatient care. Central to the assessment process is the cross-validation of the patient's report of trauma exposure and PTSD symptoms with evidence of combat exposure in the veteran's military records. Postmilitary symptomatology should be cross-checked for consistency with the report of the patient's significant others. Reports of nightmares and sleep disturbance can be validated by the observations of nurses on the night shift.

Although the relationship between the cognitive processing of trauma-related stimuli and concurrent physiological arousal is not fully delineated by current research, psychophysiological assessment can provide additional information, which may be useful when integrated with other assessment data. The main point is that the clinician needs to be aware of the potential influence of secondary gain factors and to rule these out aggressively prior to treatment. The motivation for financial compensation is related to a payoff for continued illness and may become a disincentive for therapeutic change. It can contaminate the treatment of even legitimate cases of PTSD. The detection of secondary gain interests does not necessarily indicate malingering. Patients may have significant PTSD problems and may also be seeking compensation. Nevertheless, the reward for remaining ill in such cases may outweigh the desire for therapeutic change and thus may adversely influence treatment efforts.

Expectancy Considerations

Prior to initiating treatment, it is always beneficial to discuss what can and cannot be realistically expected as potential outcomes of inpatient hospitalization. Many patients who come to the hospital for treatment of PTSD have developed the belief that treatment can completely turn their lives around before they are discharged. Although treatment efforts may reduce the level of subjective distress and start a patient on the road to rehabilitation, it needs to be made clear that a successful outcome requires a long-term perspective. The inpatient phase of treatment is the first step of a healing process that requires time, outpatient follow-up, and an active role on the part of the patient. The evaluation of the patient's expectancies regarding treatment, and educational efforts to correct unrealistically high goals, are crucial and should be considered as early as possible after the patient is admitted. An early effort in this regard may prove important during the later stages of treatment if the patient becomes dissatisfied with progress and discovers that there is no "magic wand" to erase all clinical problems. An emphasis on a long-term perspective of therapeutic gain and the need for active participation by the patient in the process can greatly assist clinical efforts to address trauma-related psychological problems: Fostering realistic expectations on the part of the patient is likely to promote the motivation for long-term treatment adherence.

Assessment

General Considerations

The initial purpose of assessment in cases of suspected combat-related PTSD is to make diagnostic determinations about PTSD and possible competing or coexisting disorders. Subsequent purposes include identifying target symptoms and establishing an ongoing treatment evaluation process. Current behavioral conceptualizations of PTSD incorporate Mowrer's (1960) two-factor theory to account for the conditioned emotional reactivity and avoidance so often seen in the disorder (Foy, Osato, Houskamp, & Neumann, in press). Thus, behavioral assessment methods for combat-related PTSD resemble those already in use with other anxiety disorders.

Since assessment and treatment are inseparable elements in a behavioral approach, identification and ongoing evaluation of PTSD-related target behaviors are critical components. Use of a three-channel response-monitoring system to track relevant overt behaviors, cognitions, and autonomic reactions is needed for PTSD assessment, as it is for assessment of other types of anxiety disorders. However, behavioral strategies for assessing combat-related PTSD must also take into account the many differences between this debilitating, chronic disorder and other less severe forms of anxiety disorder. For example, trauma exposure in combat often consists of terrible episodic events occurring over an extended period of time. This exposure to chronic threat may elicit extreme forms of coping and adaptation. Accordingly, assessment efforts need to be geared to the high probability of comorbidity with other disorders, such as substance abuse, depression, and panic disorder.

The prevalence of Axis II disorders, especially antisocial and borderline types, may be as high as 30–40% in the population of Vietnam veterans served by VA Medical Centers. However, there is reason for caution in making a concurrent Axis II diagnosis. Axis II diagnosis carries the implication of lifelong dysfunction and can serve to reinforce the negative opinions of some clinical staff members that character disorder must have preceded trauma exposure. Importantly, recent findings from studies of antisocial personality disorder and combat-related PTSD show that preadult antisocial characteristics do not significantly relate to development of PTSD. However, these studies do show that high combat exposure, even in the absence of preadult antisocial characteristics, is significantly related to presence of adult antisocial characteristics (Resnick, Foy, Donahoe, & Miller, 1989; Barrett, Resnick, Foy, Flanders, & Stroup, 1989).

These considerations notwithstanding, coping strategies that have the appearance of Axis II disorders are maladaptive and merit clinical attention in their own right. We are not suggesting that clinical management strategies for PTSD patients who also have characterological features differ from the principles that would be used with lifelong Axis II cases. However, staff attitudes toward the patients may well need to be examined carefully, lest implicit negative biases against patients presenting long-standing character pathology become unacknowledged but influential factors in the treatment environment.

In a medical center setting, patients are referred from either "hot" or "cold" sources. A "hot" referral comes from a familiar clinical source that can provide reliable historical and assessment information. Examples of this kind of referral are those made by Vet Centers or by other medical center treatment teams or units. A patient will have already been "worked up" to the point at which a referral for more specialized PTSD-related assessment and treatment is indicated. In the case of a "cold" referral, the patient is referred directly from an initial screening in an admissions and evaluations unit of the medical center to the PTSD program. Under these circumstances, very little information may be available about the patient initially.

The immediate advantages presented by the "hot" referral are obvious. However, it is strongly recommended that each patient be approached from the perspective that an independent evaluation is necessary, regardless of the general credibility of the clinical network that has produced the referral.

Assessment Procedures

Behavioral assessment for combat-related PTSD focuses upon two issues: trauma exposure and related psychological distress or symptoms. Common elements in behavioral assessment of combat veterans include clinical interviewing; psychosocial history; psychological tests; behavioral and physiological reactivity assessment; and archival information review. In actual practice, a stepwise approach will include a combination of these procedures to elicit multimodal information about patients' trauma exposure and their current psychological functioning.

The clinical interview serves to gather initial diagnostic information, including a client's description of current psychological distress and details of the traumatic experience(s). Under ideal circumstances, information obtained by clinical interview will serve as a primary element in establishing a PTSD diagnosis on the basis of expert professional judgment. However, in cases where the clinician lacks extensive experience in the assessment of trauma victims, a structured diagnostic interview approach may be used. There are now several instruments available; of these, the Structured Clinical Interview for DSM-III-R (Spitzer & Williams, 1986) and the Diagnostic Interview Schedule (Robins, Helzer, & Croughan, 1981) are most widely used.

Taking a thorough psychosocial history is necessary in order to assess a veteran's level of pretrauma adjustment. In addition, information can be obtained regarding other risk–resiliency factors that may mediate the relationship between trauma exposure and distress. Modalities through which historical information can be obtained include the veteran's self-report, reports from significant others, and archival sources. In order to enlist their consent and cooperation in obtaining this information, patients are told that it is important for the treatment team to get to know them as persons before, during, and after their military experiences. In this context, the need to contact other first-degree relatives is easily presented and accepted. As a general rule, a person selected as a collateral informant needs to have had frequent contact with a patient throughout the time frame of interest. We have used the strategy of contacting siblings who grew up in the same family environment to serve as collateral informants about a patient's family and developmental history. One efficient method of obtaining this information is to use the premilitary section of the Vietnam Veterans History Questionnaire (VVHQ; Foy, Sipprelle, Rueger, & Carroll, 1984) for a collateral informant's responses to the same questions answered by the patient. The information thus obtained provides the means for a direct comparison of data from two independent sources.

Use of a structured self-report questionnaire to obtain pretrauma data is both systematic and efficient, in that many veterans can complete the questionnaire on their own, which saves therapy time for other tasks. We have used the VVHQ in combat-related cases for several years (Foy et al., 1984) and are currently using modified versions in cases of gang-related violence, sexual assault, and domestic violence. This instrument provides indices that can be scored for psychosocial adjustment during premilitary, military, and postmilitary time frames. For each index, data are collected for family stability, school/vocational achievement, socioeconomic status, drug and alcohol use, and disciplinary and legal problems. In addition, the VVHQ contains a combat exposure scale and a 43-item symptom checklist, which provide preliminary information on level and type of combat exposure and PTSD diagnostic status.

Several psychological tests are currently in wide use for PTSD assessment purposes. These include the Minnesota Multiphasic Personality Inventory (MMPI; Hathaway & McKinley, 1951) and the Impact of Event Scale (IES; Horowitz, Wilner, & Alvarez, 1979). In addition, symptom rating scales based on DSM-III-R criteria for PTSD are often used (e.g., Foy et al., 1984; Keane, Wolfe, & Taylor, 1987). All three types of tests can be useful in establishing a probability estimate for a PTSD diagnosis, since sensitivity and specificity rates are available for each (Litz, Penk, Gerardi, & Keane, in press). The IES and symptom rating scales are especially useful in providing continuous measures of target behaviors or symptoms for monitoring across treatment phases. A cautionary note, however, is in order regarding the use of self-report psychological tests as primary diagnostic measures: These instruments are not foolproof. The symptoms of PTSD have been widely publicized, and the face validity of some of these tests is obvious. Coached patients could easily identify diagnostic items and selectively respond to the test. More frequently in the medical center setting, patients respond with a "cry for help" response bias, in which most test items are endorsed to indicate extreme distress. In such cases, PTSD diagnostic items will be positive, as will diagnostic items for other disorders. This underscores the need for the integration of assessment information from a variety of sources in making a diagnostic determination.

Assessment of behavioral and physiological reactivity is relatively well advanced in the study of combat-related PTSD, with many reports now available (e.g., Blanchard, Kolb, Taylor, & Whittrock, 1989; Malloy, Fairbank, & Keane, 1983). These demonstrate multiple-channel assessment of reactivity to traumatic stimuli in auditory and/or visual presentation modalities. Actual presentation of trauma-related stimuli is now an accepted element of comprehensive assessment for combat survivors. However, similar assessments have yet to be reported from the study of other trauma survivors, despite the fact that exposure-based treatment methods are already being used (Foy, Resnick, Carroll, & Osato, 1990). Application of this assessment strategy to the study of other trauma survivors will provide an empirical basis for using or not using exposure treatment techniques with these populations. It may also establish a method for monitoring treatment response within and across sessions.

For the present, however, physiological assessment of combat-related PTSD is primarily an adjunctive diagnostic measure to be used along with other methods. Physiological assessment accurately identifies only two-thirds of those cases that have been positively diagnosed by other means. Thus, while its specificity (correct identification of "true-negative" cases) is high, physiological assessment has unacceptably poor sensitivity (correct identification of "true-positive" cases). This limitation means that it cannot be used as a primary means of diagnosing PTSD.

Archival record review as an evaluation strategy is especially important in cases where there may be obvious gain derived from establishing trauma victim status and a related PTSD diagnosis. For combat-related cases, examination of the veteran's release-from-active-duty form (Form DD-214) is an essential element in the verification of reported high combat exposure. In addition, the veteran's personal military file (C file) and hospital or clinic records of previous treatment are valuable archival sources for cross-validation of current self-reported historical information. Equivalent archival sources may be helpful in noncombat applications. Obviously, assessment information must be obtained from several independent sources in order to achieve the best possible "level of product" in the diagnosis and case formulation.

Figure 3.1 demonstrates the diagnostic process that occurs in the early phase of treatment for combat-related PTSD. Decisions about diagnoses and treatment options need to be made by the treatment team on an empirical basis, according to decision rules developed as primary guidelines. These criteria can also be correlated with treatment participation and outcome data, so that the treatment program can be empirically evaluated. In some cases, specialized psychological assessment of depression, social support, stressful life events, marital distress, and current family functioning may be needed. Instruments that we have found useful include the Beck Depression Inventory (Beck, Ward, Mendelson, Mock, & Erbaugh, 1961), the Social Support Questionnaire and the Life Events Survey (Sarason, Johnson, & Siegel, 1978; Sarason, Levine, Basham, & Sarason, 1983), the Family Environment Scale (Moos & Moos, 1981), and the Dyadic Adjustment Scale (Spanier, 1976).

Treatment

In our previous work describing behavioral treatment methods for PTSD, we have made distinctions between types according to the primary goal of intervention (Foy et al., 1990). Accordingly, exposure

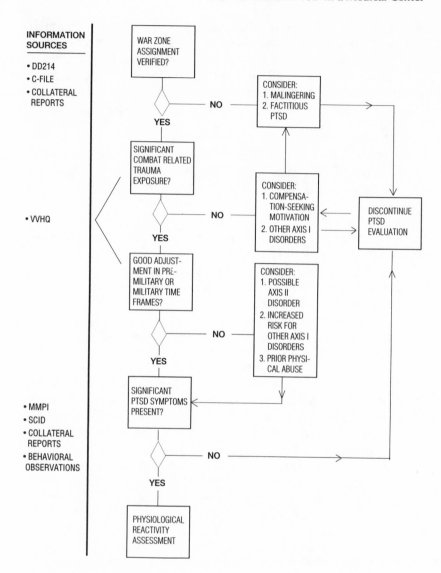

FIGURE 3.1.   Diagnostic assessment procedures for combat-related PTSD.

strategies are employed in the reduction of intrusive memories, flashbacks, and nightmares related to the original traumatic experience(s). Cognitive restructuring strategies are designed to deal with problems of meaning attributed to traumatic experiences, or related associations and assumptions that are maladaptive. Finally, skills training strategies are oriented toward teaching coping skills that either reduce personal distress or provide additional means of meeting interpersonal demands.

Exposure strategies include systematic desensitization, flooding, and implosive therapy. These techniques are used to treat the positive symptoms of PTSD, which are characterized by their intrusive and recurrent presence. Flashbacks, nightmares, and exaggerated startle responses are common examples. An imaginal modality for presentation of feared stimuli is used primarily in the treatment of combat veterans, although actual combat sights and sounds are often used in systematic pretreatment assessment procedures. In most reports, 10–15 exposure trials are used to reduce conditioned emotional arousal to traumatic cues. Treatment sessions typically last 60–120 minutes and are held once or twice weekly.

Flooding

Recent studies of direct exposure therapy in treating combat-related PTSD provide evidence for (1) incremental benefit of flooding beyond hospital milieu treatment alone (Boudewyns & Hyer, 1990; Cooper & Clum, 1989; Keane, Fairbank, Caddell, & Zimering, 1989), and (2) positive prognostic significance of physiological reactivity to traumatic cues (Boudewyns & Hyer, 1990; Mueser, Yarnold, & Foy, 1991). Thus, there is empirical support for the use of flooding as therapy for chronic combat-related PTSD in the context of hospital milieu treatment.

RATIONALE

A common-sense rationale for the use of flooding is provided. The patient is told that painful experiences must be dealt with psychologically in order for healing to occur. Those memories that have not been worked through are connected to many reminders of the experience. When these reminders occur, painful memories of the original experience are activated. The veteran has learned to stop the pain by escaping or avoiding these reminders. However, the patient now lives in fear of both the painful memories and the reminders, and his life is hemmed in by them. Flooding is described as a procedure whereby an individual can re-experience the painful memories in a safe place where it is permissible for the feared emotional reactions to occur. The potential benefit is that it may be possible to reduce the reactivity to the painful memories so that the veteran is less fearful of them. In this way, the veteran may regain control, rather than continuing to be controlled by PTSD symptoms.

CRITICAL ISSUES

Factors to be considered before flooding treatment is selected include a patient's physical condition, his personal choice for the treatment, and positive physiological assessment results (Litz, Blake, Gerardi, & Keane, 1990). Significant cardiovascular disease or risk warrants exclusion from the treatment. Also, it needs to be used only with those patients who can give informed consent for their participation. Given the negative results of two recent studies of flooding with veterans who did not show physiological reactivity to traumatic cues, the use of the procedure with nonreactive patients merits careful consideration in cost–benefit terms. If a decision is made to proceed, it is recommended that treatment be conducted under an institutionally approved research protocol. This recommendation is made not because of any known special risk under this circumstance, but rather to ensure that data are systematically collected for continuing scientific feedback on the use of the technique with physiological "nonresponders."

Although specific details of flooding treatment vary according to the stylistic preferences of the therapist and the particular needs of each patient, there are consistencies in the application of the technique. Accordingly, we have developed a set of procedures by which flooding is implemented with individual veterans.

PROCEDURAL STEPS IN PREPARATION FOR FLOODING TREATMENT

1.   The therapist must arrange the physical environment so that it is secure and comfortable. "Security" in this context means that the therapy room is soundproofed from outside noises and that the therapist has made certain that no interruptions will occur during the sessions. The room needs to be comfortably lit and temperature-controlled. It is equipped with a recliner chair that is adjusted according to the patient's preference. The therapist's standard equipment includes a heart rate monitor, chronometer, and response monitoring forms. "Subjective

units of distress" (SUDs) represent the patient's self-rating of current psychological discomfort on a scale of 0 ("no discomfort") to 10 ("highest discomfort"). Monitoring sheets are constructed so that heart rate and SUDs can be recorded according to time and phase within the treatment session.

2.   The therapist should attach and demonstrate the use of the heart rate monitor and SUDs rating sheet. He or she should allow several minutes for the patient to become comfortable in the setting, and answer any questions about the equipment or assessment procedures.

3.   The therapist begins by asking the veteran to give a description of the "memorable" events that happened during his tour of combat duty. These memories can include significant positive events or actions, as well as those "terrible" or traumatic experiences that will be the focus of flooding treatment. If the patient has trouble recalling or relating his experiences, the therapist can provide help by calling his attention to key events, such as his arrival "in country," his first firefight, or his first encounter with war-related death. This history-taking activity continues until all such events are covered.

4.   If the veteran has several traumatic events, a scene hierarchy is constructed by rank-ordering scenes according to the SUDs ratings assigned by the patient to each event or scene.

5.   The therapist then negotiates with the patient about the scene that will be used to begin flooding. Many patients will elect to start with the highest-rated scene, in hopes that success with the most difficult task will spread to less distressing scenes. Others will choose to begin with a scene lower on the hierarchy. However, since it is important for each veteran to remain in control of this choice, the therapist needs to respect it, regardless of whether it corresponds with his or her own preferences.

6.   A 15- to 20-minute scene, or "story," is constructed to serve as the starting point in the self-flooding procedure. This work is accomplished by the veteran's providing the details and the therapist's helping as necessary with prompts and questions to structure the scene. The scene is composed of three elements: the immediate antecedent situation, the actual traumatic event, and the immediate consequential reactions and events. The description needs to be as complete in detail as possible, although the first memories recalled often seem to serve as initial links for chaining memories of more obscure details that surface in later sessions.

7.   The therapist contracts with the client (a) to conduct at least eight flooding sessions, each composed of two trials over the traumatic scene; and (b) to evaluate at the end of the eight sessions whether to continue flooding the first scene, and whether to use other scenes.

PROCEDURAL STEPS IN FLOODING
TREATMENT SESSIONS

1. A self-flooding procedure is used in which the patient tells the
15- to 20-minute "story" with vivid imagery and rich detail across sensory modalities, including sights, sounds, and smells.

2. The *therapist's role* is to provide prompts, questions, and encouragement as needed to help the veteran stay on task. The goal is to
elicit the conditioned emotional response by having the veteran tell all
details of the "story" without obviously omitting details or rushing
through the scene to avoid contact with the painful emotions attached to
it.

3. The therapist monitors and records heart rate at regular
intervals (e.g., 30 seconds) to (a) ensure that the patient experiences
continuous exposure to highly arousing scene elements; and (b) provide
a record of autonomic responses over the course of the treatment
session.

4. Treatment sessions are staged so that approximate time allotments for heart rate monitoring are as follows:

a. Pretreatment: 2 minutes
b. Flooding trial 1:   20 minutes
c. Intertrial interval: 5 minutes
d. Flooding trial 2:   20 minutes
e. Posttreatment: 5 minutes

5. For organization and monitoring purposes each session is
composed of five phases, as noted in the list above. The pretreatment
phase allows the veteran to adapt to the treatment setting and provides
baseline heart rate and SUDs measures. The flooding trials are intended
to elicit sustained maximal arousal in the presence of traumatic cues, so
that habituation occurs within trials and extinction of arousal occurs
over treatment sessions. The intertrial interval and posttreatment phases
are intended to provide a time for stabilization of SUDs and heart rate, so
that the next phase begins or the session terminates with autonomic activity and distress at comfortable levels.

6. The therapist should record patient SUDs ratings at least once
per phase.

7. The time allotments listed above are estimations that are not
ironclad. Time adjustments will be needed in order to accomplish the
purposes of the phases.

IMPLEMENTATION DIFFICULTIES

Although the preceding procedural steps may give the appearance of being "cut and dried" in their application, in actual practice adjustments will be needed to accommodate the situation and needs of the individual veteran. Two commonly encountered problems are difficulties in obtaining clear imagery and avoidance of the re-exposure task in the self-flooding procedure. Patients may also fear that they will lose control during a session, causing embarrassment, physical harm to themselves or the therapist, or property damage.

In the case of imagery problems, it is useful to assess imagery clarity across sensory modalities. The veteran's abilities to imagine sights, sounds, smells and bodily sensations may be differentially affected. "Subjective units of imagery" can be assessed for each sensory modality by asking the patient to give a rating from 0 ("unclear") to 10 ("very clear") for a particular scene. The therapist can use "sensory prompts" (e.g., "What are you seeing? hearing? smelling?") at the outset of flooding. It can be helpful to use the metaphor of tuning a TV or radio to improve the veteran's visual image clarity.

Difficulties with avoidance can take several forms. Perhaps the most obvious avoidant behavior is engaging in nonemergency "no-shows" for scheduled sessions after agreeing to undertake the procedure. It is recommended that this type of avoidance be managed by renegotiating the contract with the veteran to begin flooding only when he informs the therapist that he is now ready to begin. A second type of avoidance is the presentation of unrelated material in the therapy session that displaces the flooding procedure. In the case of nonurgent issues, the therapist needs to remind the patient of the agreed-upon therapy task and bring the session back to the flooding procedure. If necessary, sessions can be structured so that the veteran's wishes to discuss other urgent clinical issues can be honored by allowing a brief period for that purpose before flooding.

Still another type of task-avoidant behavior is the use of emotional distancing, distraction, or inattention during the actual self-flooding task. More accurately, this represents "escape responding" in learning terms. The therapist's task in this situation is to remind the veteran that his complete involvement in the scene is needed in order for the flooding task to be accomplished. Although the patient may control his distress in this way in the short term, the probable effect on the course of flooding treatment is to prolong it. The therapist needs to provide encouragement empathically, but firmly, for full participation in the self-flooding.

The patient's fears of losing control are acknowledged, and reassurance about the self-guided nature of the flooding procedure is provided. The therapist needs to inform the veteran that such episodes are rare, but if the emotional intensity becomes too great, the patient is free (and the therapist will help him) to take a break, and treatment will resume only when he indicates that he is ready.

Cognitive Restructuring

Cognitive restructuring methods are used to deal with troublesome issues related to patients' appraisals of their traumatic experiences. Cognitive distortions can affect an individual's ability to evaluate both external factors (such as threat) and personal factors (such as resources and coping skills). Cognitive restructuring can be applied under either or both of two conditions. First, it can be used to correct misattributions of causality and responsibility associated with remembered traumatic scenes. This can be done in conjunction with exposure therapy immediately following exposure trials over the traumatic scene.

A second alternative is that cognitive restructuring can be done independently in individual therapy sessions devoted primarily to that task. In actual practice, a combination of the two strategies is often used: Restructuring of a specific trauma is done in conjunction with flooding, whereas addressing the veteran's world view is accomplished in sessions devoted to that task.

Basic life assumptions that may be altered by traumatic victimization include the invulnerability of the self, the meaningfulness and equitability of life, and positive self-esteem in life experiences (Janoff-Bulman, 1985). These implicit assumptions or cognitive schemas serve the individual by allowing "automatic" psychological functioning, in which these needs are assumed to be met without requiring evaluation of each environment and situation. However, these key assumptions may be shattered or polarized by the experience of traumatic victimization, so that extreme fearfulness, mistrust, and self-blame become prominent. Through an explicit review of the veteran's life assumptions both before and after the traumatic experience, the patient is empowered by acknowledgment of these fundamental assumptions and gains the choice of moderating extreme reactions in favor of a more balanced perspective. The therapist's role is that of assisting the patient in the discovery of these implicit assumptions, thereby making them explicit and modifiable.

Other key cognitive elements in cognitive restructuring include foreseeability, controllability, and culpability. "Foreseeability" refers to whether the occurrence of a catastrophic event could have realistically been anticipated in advance. "Controllability" refers to the extent to which a traumatic outcome could have been modified through human actions. Similarly, "culpability" refers to the extent to which the actions or inactions of particular persons were directly implicated in the outcome of a tragic event.

PROCEDURAL STEPS IN ASSESSMENT FOR COGNITIVE RESTRUCTURING OF SPECIFIC TRAUMATIC MEMORIES

1. During the patient's description of the traumatic scene(s), the therapist records critical junctures in the scenario that led to the ultimate traumatic outcome. These are "decision points," apparent in retrospect, at which the choice of a different course of action might have changed the ultimate outcome.

2. If the veteran's description of the scene(s) does not include obvious references to critical junctures, the therapist gently poses these as possibilities. The patient's implicit assumptions about foreseeability and controllability of the ultimate outcome are noted as they are reflected in the veteran's narrative of each critical juncture. The patient's assumptions about human culpability for events leading to the ultimate outcome—his own culpability, as well as that of others—are also noted. When critical junctures in the traumatic scene(s) have been identified and the patient's assumptions for each have been assessed in terms of foreseeability, controllability, and culpability, active cognitive restructuring can begin.

PROCEDURAL STEPS IN COGNITIVE RESTRUCTURING OF SPECIFIC MEMORIES

1. Critical junctures in the traumatic scene(s) are addressed consecutively. For each juncture, the therapist elicits clarifying statements and information from the veteran, so that assumptions that have been implicit (and perhaps even unknown to the patient) become explicit and are personally "claimed."

2. Once the patient's assumptions have been made explicit, the therapist and veteran form a team whose purpose is to examine carefully each critical juncture. The aim is to assess realistic alternative courses of

action for each critical juncture, given "reasonable" assessments of foreseeability and controllability.

3.   Differences are then noted between the patient's personal assumptions and the findings of the examination conducted by the therapist–veteran team. Cognitive restructuring then proceeds with the patien'st examining each difference and making a choice about a new (or reaffirmed) formulation of critical junctures in the traumatic event(s).

4.   The veteran then restructures the event by formulating a narrative version of the experience that reflects a reasoned processing and personal acceptance of its occurrence and importance in the patient's life.

5.   Thought stopping and guided self-dialogue are specific techniques that are applied as necessary to interrupt and replace old thinking associated with the traumatic memory in its unprocessed form.

PROCEDURAL STEPS IN ASSESSMENT FOR COGNITIVE RESTRUCTURING OF THE VETERAN'S WORLD VIEW

1.   The therapist begins assessment by conceptually framing the veteran's life into premilitary, military, and postmilitary periods. The therapist should elicit detailed personal history regarding family, school and social involvements, in order to discover the patient's implicit core assumptions about physical and psychological invulnerability, life's meaning and equitability, and self-worth as reflected in life experiences.

2.   The therapist determines whether the premilitary history includes *early trauma exposure* such as physical or sexual abuse. For those veterans whose premilitary experience included traumatic victimization, that trauma experience becomes the focus for eliciting information about psychological reactions and changes in life assumptions. If no premilitary trauma exposure is indicated, then the combat-related trauma becomes the focal event.

PROCEDURAL STEPS IN COGNITIVE RESTRUCTURING OF THE VETERAN'S WORLD VIEW

1.   The therapist begins the restructuring process by eliciting the patient's rationale for entering the military at the particular time he did so and for choosing the particular branch of the service that he chose. In the case of those who were drafted into service, the rationale for waiting

to be drafted rather than enlisting to avoid the draft is explored. For those who enlisted, reasons for choosing the branch of service, other contractual conditions of service, and training options selected are explored. The therapist needs to pay particular attention to the veteran's implicit assumptions about predictability and controllability of ultimate outcome, as reflected in the narrative about entering service. This may be an early critical juncture in the patient's memory representation of combat-related trauma.

2.   For those veterans with a previous trauma history, information about how the earlier trauma was processed is elicited. Changes in core life assumptions are noted, and the relationship between prior trauma experience and expectations for military service is explored. In some cases, individuals entered the service hoping to be rescued from earlier victimization experiences and their consequences. The first clinical task of restructuring is to make explicit these previously implicit assumptions about what military service was expected to accomplish.

3.   Military service is conceptually divided into precombat, combat, and postcombat periods. Critical personal experiences over the course of military service and related changes in life assumptions are elicited and explored. The veteran's perception of preparation for combat is elicited, and the first signs of perceived victimization in the patient's narrative are noted.

4.   Information is elicited about the veteran's adaptation to a life-threatening environment. Details are obtained regarding what the patient did psychologically and physically in order to survive. The veteran's revised world view in the combat situation is explored and reframed, if necessary, as a positive adaptation to a life-threatening situation. Details about how the patient's assignment to the war zone ended are elicited, so that perceptions of differences between a life-threatening environment and military assignment outside the war zone are obtained.

5.   Postcombat military experiences are reviewed. The veteran's assessment of personal adjustment to service assignments following combat is solicited, and evidence of life assumptions reflecting victimization during combat is noted. Information about the patient's discharge from active duty and transition into civilian life is obtained.

6.   The veteran's view of postmilitary adjustment in light of the previous traumatic experience(s) is elicited. Evidence for continuation of life assumptions better fitted to a life-threatening combat environment is noted.

7.   On the basis of the patient's evolving life assumptions as reflected in the review conducted in the first six steps, a question is posed regarding the adequacy of the veteran's continuing to hold on to extreme

assumptions better suited for a combat (or survival) situation. Reformulation of current life assumptions toward a "sadder, but wiser" posture is then undertaken.

Skills Training Approaches

Skills training approaches represent a third type of behavioral strategy
for treating PTSD and related interpersonal difficulties. These techniques include relaxation training, anger management, problem-solving
skills, assertion training, and family or dyadic communication skills
training. These can be used as discrete methods, but they are probably
used more often as adjunctive to or in combination with other methods.

One area in which PTSD studies have identified a particular need
for a skills training approach is that of marital/family discord, which is
often found in conjunction with chronic PTSD (Carroll, Rueger, Foy, &
Donahoe, 1985). Communication in intimate relationships may become
dysfunctional when one of the individuals is victimized through the experience of trauma. Education about predictable reactions to overwhelming experiences is important for the victim and other family
members (Carroll, Foy, Cannon, & Zwier, 1991). Communication skills
training can be used to promote the initially painful but necessary disclosure of the traumatic experience by survivors to their partners. Corre-
spondingly, the spouse or partner's active listening skills can also be
targeted, so that the survivor's tendency to avoid topics, activities, and
emotions associated with the trauma is not inadvertently reinforced.

In addition, relapse prevention skills have recently been high-
lighted as critical for many patients with combat-related PTSD who
show comorbidity for substance abuse disorders. Abueg and Fairbank
(in press) have developed a structured skills approach for training patients in the use of these strategies to reduce the risk of relapse into substance abuse. Preliminary treatment outcome results for this approach
appear promising.

Clinical Predictors of Treatment Outcome

Inpatient treatment can help reduce the intrusive positive symptoms of
PTSD (e.g., flashbacks, traumatic memories, nightmares) in an environment providing support and crisis management. In addition, interventions focused on cognitive factors and skill-building needs can be
initiated during a period of inpatient clinical care. However, the long-
term efficacy of treatment for PTSD depends considerably upon the

quality of aftercare. Chronic combat-related PTSD is a severe type of anxiety disorder that often presents with multiple concomitant psychiatric problems. Treatment planning is best conceptualized as a long-term process that will include short-term, intensive treatment of acute symptoms and long-term follow-up and rehabilitation. Accordingly, important predictors of treatment success are (1) the patient's motivation to engage in a long-term rehabilitation process requiring sustained treatment adherence and (2) the availability of adequate clinical resources.

Treatment generalizability from an inpatient setting to the veteran's community situation is a critical component of long-term efficacy in most psychiatric disorders, and PTSD is no exception. The patient's return to the community is accompanied by the return of social, work, and general life stressors that can undo any gains made in the medical center setting. To help remedy generalizability problems, it is important to educate the patient during hospitalization about the probability of such problems, and to promote the patient's adherence to an outpatient and/or support group aftercare plan. Any expectations that the patient may hold regarding a "quick fix" in the hospital need to be identified and addressed as soon as possible. A realistic attitude toward what can be achieved in the medical center setting and what will need to be a part of aftercare treatment will help promote treatment adherence after discharge. Also, educational effort about the treatment process will help defuse angry and bitter reactions when patients learn that the hospital cannot provide a "magic wand" for the quick cure of chronic PTSD and related adjustment problems.

Obviously, promoting generalizability of treatment results through the use of aftercare follow-up requires that sufficient clinical resources be available to the veteran. Fortunately, there are more clinical resources available to combat veterans today than there were 10 years ago. Most urban areas have Vet Centers, which provide daily support groups and may also provide counseling services for spouses and other family members. Most VA Medical Centers offer a variety of outpatient services that can be useful in maintaining inpatient treatment gains. Individual and group modalities can often be found that focus on marital and family assistance, the promotion of coping and problem-solving skills, and cognitive restructuring.

The needs of veterans who experience exacerbated PTSD symptoms or sizable readjustment problems have been successfully addressed at some VA Medical Centers through short-term "stabilization units." Such units are not geared to in-depth, trauma resolution, but are oriented toward problem solving strategies aimed at the specific difficulties that patients encounter in the community. The goals are rehabilitation and increased coping skills; the most frequent targets are problems with anger management, communication skills, depression, self-esteem, and social isolation. The patient may return for periodic stabilization on an "as-needed" basis.

Other predictors of long-term treatment success or failure should be mentioned. The severity of the patient's PTSD symptomatology and the extent of comorbidity are strongly related to long-term outcome. For example, the research and clinical literature on PTSD is replete with evidence of the high prevalence of alcohol abuse among Vietnam veterans with trauma-related problems. The co-occurrence of these problems should alert the clinician to the increased risk for postdischarge relapse and the need for careful aftercare planning. Although the relationship between PTSD and alcohol abuse can be understood in terms of self-medication, the etiological factors contributing to the frequent association may be more complex. Both clinical disorders share a pervasive pattern of avoidance as a characteristic coping style. As a result, substance abuse not only may provide short-term relief of subjective distress, but may also strengthen and reinforce inclinations toward long-term problem avoidance and poor psychosocial adaptation. Thus, the presence of a dual diagnosis for a PTSD patient should indicate to the treatment team that the veteran is a member of a high-risk population. Aftercare treatment planning will need to consider the high probability of avoidant behavior and treatment nonadherence.

In sum, the provision of problem-specific aftercare and the promotion of treatment adherence have been emphasized as critical components of successful treatment generalization and maintenance. Careful attention to postdischarge treatment planning is especially important for PTSD patients who are at high risk for relapse. Those patients who evidence clinically significant comorbidity are examples of such a high-risk population. The development of effective treatment strategies for PTSD patients with dual diagnoses is a task worthy of considerably more research attention and clinical innovation. At present, unfortunately, the most common treatment approach for PTSD patients with multiple clinical problems is piecemeal, focused on one problem in isolation from others. The formulation of multifaceted interventions that address the simultaneous and interactive nature of comorbidity problems has thus far been limited. An expanded conceptual focus would probably be very beneficial in terms of reduced relapse rates and improved long-term treatment efficacy.

References

Abueg, F. R., & Fairbank, J. A. (in press). Behavioral treatment of the PTSD–substance abuser: A multidimensional stage model. In P. A. Saigh (Ed.), *Posttraumatic stress disorder: Behavioral assessment and treatment*. Elmsford, NY: Maxwell Press.

Barrett, D. B., Resnick, H. S., Foy, D. W., Flanders, W. D., & Stroup, N. E. (1989, August). *Antisocial behavior and posttraumatic stress disorder in Vietnam veterans*. Paper presented at the annual convention of the American Psychological Association, New Orleans.

Beck, A. T., Ward, C. H., Mendelson, M., Mock, J., & Erbaugh, J. (1961). An inventory for measuring depression. *Archives of General Psychiatry, 4,* 561–571.

Berman, S., Price, S., & Gusman, F. D. (1982). An inpatient program for Vietnam combat veterans in a Veterans Administration hospital. *Hospital and Community Psychiatry, 42,* 115–119.

Blanchard, E. B., Kolb, L. C., Taylor, A. E., & Whittrock, D. A. (1989). Cardiac response to relevant stimuli as an adjunct in diagnosing posttraumatic stress disorder: Replication and extension. *Behavior Therapy, 20,* 535–543.

Boudewyns, P. A., & Hyer, L. (1990). Physiologic response to combat memories and preliminary treatment outcome in Vietnam veteran PTSD patients treated with direct therapeutic exposure. *Behavior Therapy, 21,* 63–87.

Carroll, E. M., Foy, D. W., Cannon, B. J., & Zwier, G. (1991). Assessment issues involving the families of trauma victims. *Journal of Traumatic Stress, 4,* 25–40.

Carroll, E. M., Rueger, D. B., Foy, D. W., & Donahoe, C. P. (1985). Vietnam combat veterans with posttraumatic stress disorder: Analysis of marital and cohabiting adjustment. *Journal of Abnormal Psychology, 94,* 329–337.

Cooper, N. A., & Clum, G. A. (1989). Imaginal flooding as a supplementary treatment for PTSD in combat veterans: A controlled study. *Behavior Therapy, 20,* 381–391.

Foy, D. W., Osato, S. S., Houskamp, B. M., & Neumann, D. A. (in press). PTSD etiology. In P. A. Saigh (Ed.), *Posttraumatic stress disorder: Behavioral assessment and treatment*. Elmsford, NY: Maxwell Press.

Foy, D. W., Resnick, H. S., Carroll, E. M., & Osato, S. S. (1990). Behavior therapy in posttraumatic stress disorder. In M. Hersen & A. S. Bellack (Eds.), *Handbook of comparative adult treatments* (pp. 302–315). New York: Wiley.

Foy, D. W., Sipprelle, R. C., Rueger, D. B., & Carroll, E. M. (1984). Etiology of posttraumatic stress disorder in Vietnam veterans: Analysis of premilitary, military, and combat exposure influences. *Journal of Consulting and Clinical Psychology, 52,* 79–87.

Friedman, M. J. (1991). Biological approaches to the diagnosis and treatment of posttraumatic stress disorder. *Journal of Traumatic Stress, 4,* 67–91.

Hathaway, S. R., & McKinley, J. C. (1951). *MMPI manual* (rev. ed.). New York: Psychological Corp.

Horowitz, M., Wilner, N., & Alvarez, W. (1979). Impact of Event Scale: A measure of subjective stress. *Psychosomatic Medicine, 41,* 209–218.

Janoff-Bulman, R. (1985). The aftermath of victimization: Rebuilding shattered assumptions. In C. R. Figley (Ed.), *Trauma and its wake: Vol. 1. The study and treatment of posttraumatic stress disorder* (pp. 15–35). New York: Brunner/Mazel.

Keane, T. M., Fairbank, J. A., Caddell, J. A., & Zimering, R. T. (1989). Implosive (flooding) therapy reduces symptoms of PTSD in Vietnam combat veterans. *Behavior Therapy, 20,* 245–260.

Keane, T. M., Wolf, J., & Taylor, K. L. (1987). Posttraumatic stress disorder: Evidence for diagnostic validity and methods of psychological assessment. *Journal of Clinical Psychology, 43,* 32–43.

Litz, B. T., Blake, D. D., Gerardi, R. G., & Keane, T. M. (1990). Decision making guidelines for the use of direct therapeutic exposure in the treatment of posttraumatic stress disorder. *Behavior Therapy, 13,* 91–93.

Litz, B. T., Penk, W. E., Gerardi, R. J., & Keane, T. M. (in press). Assessment of posttraumatic stress disorder. In P. A. Saigh (Ed.), *Posttraumatic stress disorder: Behavioral assessment and treatment.* Elmsford, NY: Maxwell Press.

Malloy, P. F., Fairbank, J. A., & Keane, T. M. (1983). Validation of a multimethod assessment of posttraumatic stress disorders in Vietnam veterans. *Journal of Consulting and Clinical Psychology, 51,* 488–494.

Moos, R. H., & Moos, B. S. (1981). *Family Environment Scale manual.* Palo Alto, CA: Consulting Psychologists Press.

Mowrer, O. H. (1960). *Learning theory and behavior.* New York: Wiley.

Mueser, K. T., Yarnold, P. R., & Foy, D. W. (1991). Statistical analysis for single case design: Evaluating outcome of imaginal exposure treatment of chronic PTSD. *Behavior Modification, 15,* 134–155.

Resnick, H. S., Foy, D. W., Donahoe, C. P., & Miller, E. N. (1989). Antisocial behavior and posttraumatic stress disorder in Vietnam veterans. *Journal of Clinical Psychology, 45,* 820–832.

Robins, L. N., Helzer, J. E., & Croughan, J. (1981). National Institute of Mental Health Diagnostic Interview Schedule: Its history, characteristics, and validity. *Archives of General Psychiatry, 38,* 381–389.

Rosen, J., & Bohon, S. (1990). Pharmacotherapy of posttraumatic stress disorder. In M. Hersen & A. S. Bellack (Eds.), *Handbook of comparative adult treatments* (pp. 316–326). New York: Wiley.

Sarason, I. G., Johnson, J. H., & Siegel, J. (1978). Assessing the impact of life changes: Development of the Life Experiences Survey. *Journal of Consulting and Clinical Psychology, 46,* 932–946.

Sarason, I. G., Levine, H. M., Basham, R. B., & Sarason, B. R. (1983). Assessing social support: The Social Support Questionnaire. *Journal of Personality and Social Psychology, 52,* 127–139.

Spanier, G. B. (1976). Measuring dyadic adjustment: New scales for assessing the quality of marriage and similar dyads. *Journal of Marriage and the Family, 38,* 15–28.

Spitzer, R. L., & Williams, J. B. W. (1986). *Structured Clinical Interview for DSM-III-R.* New York: New York State Psychiatric Institute.

4

Assessment and Treatment of Post-Traumatic Stress Disorder among Battered Women

MARY ANN DUTTON

The psychological trauma associated with woman battering is increasingly recognized as an important component of intervention with battered women (Dutton, in press; Walker, 1984), in addition to the important issues of safety and decision making (Douglas, 1987). Problems facing abused women are not limited to their traumatic reactions to prior abuse, however, since many battered women continue to face real threats of recurring traumatic violence and abuse, even after they leave their relationships (Browne, 1987). Accordingly, many battered women who seek help from mental health professionals do so with a focus on the ongoing threat of abuse and their efforts to respond to it. Other battered women seek help long after immediate threats of abuse have passed, for psychological symptoms related to the prior abuse, some of which are characteristic of PTSD. Thus, trauma-related therapy with battered women must accommodate the breadth of their issues.

The strategy for clinical intervention with battered women presented here is a multimodal assessment and treatment approach that addresses relevant clinical issues within which the treatment of PTSD is imbedded. Similarly, Fairbank (1989) has stated that problem definition and formulation for combat veterans exhibiting symptoms of PTSD should take into account "other potential reactions to trauma, as well as problems that tend to co-occur with PTSD" (p. 305) through "multimethod, multisource approaches to assessment" (p. 304). Advocacy for safety (Schechter, 1987) and empowerment through choice making (Dutton, in press; Pence, 1987) are critical components of an overall intervention strategy for battered women.

A cognitive–behavioral theoretical foundation is used in this chapter to address assessment and treatment of PTSD as it applies to battered women. Integrated within this discussion is a feminist perspective on the social context, defined by gender and other dimensions of social oppression, within which both the problem of abuse originates and the intervention by professionals occurs.

Domestic Abuse as Trauma

Domestic abuse includes physical violence, sexual violence, and psychological abuse (Ganley, 1981, 1989; Pence & Paymar, 1986), which in some circumstances can be likened to the torture of hostages (Graham, Rawlings, & Rimini, 1988; Scrignar, 1988). Psychological abuse can include threats of further abuse—for example, threats to kill or injure the battered woman, her children, or other family members and friends; threats of sexual assault against a child; or threats of economic and financial ruin. That life-threatening events are frequently experienced by many battered women is now well established, leaving little doubt that domestic abuse constitutes "traumatic experience" as defined by current diagnostic criteria.

Effects of Domestic Abuse on Women

Psychological sequelae of traumatic experiences within intimate relationships where women face ongoing threats of physical, sexual, and psychological abuse are many and varied. This section describes those effects within three categories: (1) psychological symptoms, including those referred to as PTSD, as well as other indicators of psychological distress and dysfunction; (2) cognitive changes, including attributions and attitudes; and (3) disturbances in relationship skills beyond those used within an abusive relationship.

The most widely recognized effects of domestic abuse have been those symptoms associated with PTSD and various other indicators of psychological distress and dysfunction described in the literature. Some trauma-related symptoms may also function as coping mechanisms (e.g., avoidance), although others do not. Frequent symptom patterns that have been identified as psychological responses to domestic abuse can be summarized as follows: (1) intrusion symptoms, or re-experiencing of the traumatic experience (Dutton, Perrin, Chrestman, & Halle, 1990; Houskamp, Foy, & Baranoff, 1989); (2) avoidance symptoms, which function to reduce awareness of the traumatic experience and its aftermath (Dutton et al., 1990; Houskamp et al., 1989); (3) anxiety (Hilberman & Munson, 1978; Rosal, Dutton-Douglas, & Perrin, 1990; Trimpey, 1989), agoraphobic symptoms (Saunders, 1990), sleep disturbance, difficulty concentrating, hypervigilance, physiological reactivity, and anger or rage, all of which share a common dimension of autonomic arousal; (4) depression and grief (Campbell, 1989; Turner & Shapiro, 1986), shame, lowered self-esteem, suicide ideation, gestures, or other self-destructive behaviors; (5) somatic complaints (Jaffee, Wolfe, Wilson, & Zak, 1986; Koss, Woodruff, & Koss, 1990); (6) use of alcohol (Stark et al., 1981) and other addictive behaviors; and (7) impaired functioning in occupational and other social roles.

Changes in cognitive schemas, or basic core beliefs about the world, oneself, and others (Blackman, 1989; Foa, Steketee, & Rothbaum, 1989; Janoff-Bulman & Frieze, 1983; McCann, Sakheim, & Abrahamson, 1988), represent a second group of sequelae of domestic abuse. The specific cognitions related to the trauma of being battered include (1) loss of assumption of invulnerability or personal safety; (2) loss of view of the world as meaningful; (3) perception of futility and diminished alternatives about available options to protect oneself; (4) negative beliefs about self; (5) developing increased tolerance for abusive behavior; and (6) tolerance of the cognitive inconsistency of abuse in an intimate relationship. These cognitive changes may be associated with increased emotional distress and decreased ability to protect oneself in the abusive situation.

Relational disturbances, like psychological symptoms and cognitive changes, are considered to result from exposure to abuse. Although it is obvious that abuse would seriously disrupt any intimate relationship, there may be paradoxical effects in some cases: The victims' emotional dependency and attachment to the abusers may increase (Dutton & Painter, 1981; Graham et al., 1988).

Chronic exposure to abuse in an intimate relationship can also influence one's ability to function adequately in personal relationships other than the abusive one. Relationship skills influenced by intimate abuse include difficulty with trusting and intimacy. Difficulty with using assertiveness to set personal boundaries in nonabusive relationships (e.g., saying no to unwanted sex, expressing a preference different from that of the abuser) may generalize from the previous abusive relationship, in which doing so may have been a dangerous behavior, leading to an escalation of violence. Allowing emotional intimacy and sexual contact may represent too great a vulnerability, and thus too great a risk, for a formerly battered woman even in a subsequent relationship. When the battered woman decides to remain within a relationship in which the abuse has ceased for a period of time, relationship difficulties are even more expectable and understandable.

Model for Post-Traumatic Reactions among Battered Women

Most theoretical models of traumatic response fail to account etiologically for the array of PTSD symptomatology (Foy, Osato, Houskamp, & Neumann, in press), much less the range of other reactions to trauma, such as self-blame, lowered self-esteem, and drug and alcohol abuse.

The present discussion of post-traumatic reactions among battered women is based on a model recently presented elsewhere (Dutton, in press), which identifies abuse as the necessary and sufficient antecedent to explain individual post-traumatic reactions occurring within a social, political, economic, and cultural context. Mediating variables are offered as an means of explaining individual differences in post-traumatic response patterns, including the development of chronic PTSD. Figure 4.1 illustrates the model.

Traumatic events include both the discrete events representing acute physical, sexual, and psychological abusive episodes, and the general "state of siege" (S. Ostoff, personal communication, January 2, 1991) that many battered women experience. The pervasively threatening environment created by the abuser's subtle gestures, occasional threats, silences, alcohol or drug binges, for example, has been referred to by Walker (1984) as the "tension-building" phase in the cycle of violence.

Mediating variables are described within six categories: (1) other current life stressors (e.g., seriously ill child or parent, terminal illness or disability, sexual abuse of one's child, job stress, comorbidity of symptoms unrelated to the occurrence of prior or current abuse); (2) social support and other resources; (3) susceptibility or vulnerability factors; (4) other (positive and negative) aspects of the relationship with the abuser, apart from the occurrence of abuse; (5) personality variables, including cognitions such as attitudes, values, and beliefs; and (6) others' response to the abuse. These categories are similar to Foy et al.'s (in press) risk and resiliency factors in their PTSD etiological hypothesis.

Battered women use various strategies to escape, avoid, or survive abuse when it actually occurs (Bowker, 1983; Pagelow, 1981). These

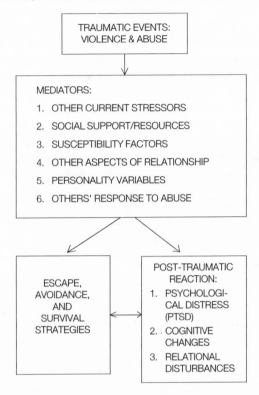

SOCIAL, CULTURAL, ECONOMIC, POLITICAL CONTEXT

TRAUMATIC EVENTS:
VIOLENCE & ABUSE

MEDIATORS:

1. OTHER CURRENT STRESSORS
2. SOCIAL SUPPORT/RESOURCES
3. SUSCEPTIBILITY FACTORS
4. OTHER ASPECTS OF RELATIONSHIP
5. PERSONALITY VARIABLES
6. OTHERS' RESPONSE TO ABUSE

ESCAPE,
AVOIDANCE,
AND
SURVIVAL
STRATEGIES

POST-TRAUMATIC
REACTION:
1. PSYCHOLOGI-
CAL DISTRESS
(PTSD)
2. . COGNITIVE
CHANGES
3. RELATIONAL
DISTURBANCES

FIGURE 4.1. Post-traumatic stress reaction model for battered women.

strategies are hypothesized both to influence and to be influenced by the post-traumatic reaction of the battered woman, and to be mediated by the variables described above.

The model describes post-traumatic reactions as (1) indicators of psychological distress, including but not limited to symptoms meeting the criteria for PTSD, as well as other problems of comorbidity related to the occurrence of abuse; (2) cognitive changes; and (3) relational disturbances. All of these types of reactions are hypothesized to result from exposure to abuse; they are also hypothesized to be interrelated, each influencing the others. In the remainder of this chapter, the focus is primarily on PTSD as a specific post-traumatic reaction to domestic abuse and violence.

Assessment

Assessment of PTSD among battered women requires a focus on each of the criteria included in the DSM-III-R (American Psychiatric Association, 1987), including (1) the traumatic event(s) or experience(s) themselves, (2) intrusion symptoms, (3) avoidance symptoms, and (4) arousal symptoms.

A number of psychometric instruments are available for the assessment of PTSD (see Watson, 1990, for a review), including structured interviews, inventory scales, and partially structured interviews and questionnaires. Many of these instruments were developed for use with combat veterans, and their utility for other populations is not yet well-established. In particular, the use of psychometric instruments for the assessment of PTSD in battered women has been noticeably absent from the literature, with few exceptions (Dutton et al.,1990; Dutton-Douglas, Perrin, Chrestman, & Faden-Strauss, 1989; Houskamp et al., 1989). Thus, this section presents an evolving approach to assessing PTSD in battered women.

Assessment of Traumatic Events: Domestic Abuse

Abuse in an intimate relationship can be approached by means of three basic methods: (1) open-ended interview, (2) structured interview, and (3) questionnaire methods (Dutton, in press). Corroborating materials (e.g., police records, medical records, prior psychotherapy records) and collateral interviews (e.g., with family members, friends, employers) are also useful in assessing the nature and extent of the abuse that has occurred. At present, a multimethod assessment strategy is recommended. The open-ended interview is useful for obtaining an initial assessment of the nature and extent of domestic abuse; it also allows the battered woman an opportunity to tell her story without the constraints imposed by a more structured format. Subsequently, the interviewer can follow up with a more structured format, identifying a specific moment-to-moment sequence of events occurring in a particular abusive episode. As if scripting a movie scene, the examiner asks about details of behavior by both the abuser and the abused in order to help develop a functional analysis of the battered woman's efforts to respond to the abuse and of post-traumatic reactions she may have experienced. The functional analysis, or "identification of important, controllable, causal functional relationships applicable to a specified set of target behaviors for an individual client" (Haynes & O'Brien, 1990, p. 654), must also take into account variables beyond those found in the immediate abuse situation, such as those identified in the model described above (e.g., the social, cultural, political, and economic context).

Finally, a variety of structured questionnaires or surveys may be used to identify the occurrence of specific abusive behaviors and their frequencies. The Conflict Tactics Scales (Straus, 1979) measure a small set of verbal and physical acts of aggression, but they do not include items referring to sexual abuse or to most types of psychological abuse. The Abusive Behavior Observation Checklist (Dutton, Freeman, & Stumpff, 1988) was developed to assess physically, sexually, and psychologically abusive behaviors experienced by battered women. It is self-administered and asks about the frequency of specific abusive behaviors and injuries within the past 12 months with the abusive partner, prior to the last 12 months with the same partner, and at any time with the current or previous partner. Tolman's (1989) Psychological Maltreatment of Women Inventory is composed of 58 items forming two empirically derived subscales: Dominance–Isolation and Emotional–Verbal Abuse. Written questionnaires eliciting information about specific abusive behaviors are useful when the goal is to develop an overall assessment of the nature of abuse to which a battered woman may have been exposed over some period of time.

Using a multidimensional strategy of assessment allows the assessor to target both the occurrence of specific abusive behaviors (structured questionnaires) and the priorities that the battered woman assigns in describing specific incidents (open-ended interview), as well as other related events surrounding the occurrence of abuse (structured interview).

Assessment of PTSD Symptoms

Assessment of symptoms of intrusion, avoidance, and arousal symptoms of PTSD can be achieved in much the same manner as for other trauma survivors. However, reports of the use of psychometric instruments to assess these PTSD criteria with battered women have to date been quite limited. Houskamp et al. (1989) used the Structured Clinical Interview for DSM-III-R (SCID; Spitzer & Williams, 1986) with battered women. A limitation of the SCID, however, is the professional level of training required for administration (Watson, 1990). The Impact of Event Scale (IES; Horowitz, Wilner, & Alvarez, 1979) has been used to assess specific intrusion and avoidance (but not arousal) symptoms of PTSD with battered women (Dutton et al., 1990; Houskamp et al.,

1989). An advantage of this 15-item scale is its ease of administration, making it desirable as a measure of outcome. The IES has been shown to correlate significantly with Keane, Malloy, and Fairbank's (1984) PTSD subscale derived from the Minnesota Multiphasic Personality Inventory (MMPI), although the correlation with the MMPI subscale was higher for the IES Avoidance subscale than the IES Intrusion subscale (Dutton-Douglas et al., 1989). Furthermore, IES scores among battered women have been found to correlate significantly with scores on the Crime-Related Post-Traumatic Stress Disorder Scale (CR-PTSD) (Dutton, Perrin, Chrestman, & Halle, 1991). (The CR-PTSD is described more fully below.)

Physiological PTSD laboratory tests have yet to become widely available (Watson, 1990) for any trauma group, and no research has yet appeared measuring physiological reactivity among battered women, although one study is currently underway in our Family Violence Program at Nova University. Although clinical reports by battered women appear to provide clear indication of physiological arousal upon exposure to abuse-relevant stimuli, more research is needed in the use of available instruments for assessing physiological arousal in PTSD among battered women.

Several psychometric instruments have been developed on the basis of empirical evidence that they effectively discriminate trauma survivors diagnosed with and without PTSD. These instruments do not assess the PTSD criteria directly, however. The MMPI subscale and the CR-PTSD are reviewed here because of the availability of data on battered women specifically.

The MMPI-derived PTSD subscale (Keane et al., 1984) was able to differentiate between four of five groups of battered women defined by their cluster membership in a cluster analysis of MMPI clinical profiles (Dutton et al., 1990). The mean PTSD subscale score was 22.7 (*SD* = 8.9) for a sample of 127 battered women with an overall range of scores from 9 to 45. Means across the five cluster groups ranged from 14.4 (*SD* = 4.2) to 36.0 (*SD*= 5.6). No study has yet validated the MMPI subscale against the DSM-III-R criteria for PTSD among battered women. Nevertheless, the results of this cluster analysis indicate some promise for use of the MMPI subscale with this population.

The CR-PTSD (Saunders, Arata, & Kilpatrick, 1990) was empirically derived from the Symptom Checklist 90—Revised (SCL-90-R) as a useful measure for classifying PTSD-positive and PTSD-negative female victims of crime; a cutoff score of .89 is employed. Using the CR-PTSD with a sample of 106 battered women seeking help from a specialized family violence clinic, Cimino (1991) found the PTSD-positive classification rate to be 60%. The CR-PTSD holds promise as a screening instrument, because of the wide use of the SCL-90-R in clinical settings.

Assessment of Other Reactions to Battering

A comprehensive assessment should include evaluation for other disorders and conditions for which battered women are at increased risk. Other sources are available describing the assessment of (1) anger (Novaco, 1979); (2) shame; (3) grief and depression (Rehm, 1988); (4) anxiety reactions, including generalized anxiety, phobic anxiety, and agoraphobic reactions (Neitzel, Bernstein, & Russell, 1988); (5) somatic complaints (Williamson, Davis, & Prather, 1988); (6) addictive behaviors (Foy, Rychtarik, & Prue, 1988); (7) shifts in cognitive schemas (McCann & Pearlman, 1990a); (8) relationship skills involving trust, intimacy, boundary setting, and traumatic bonding (Graham et al., 1988); and (9) impairment in functioning (Becker & Heimberg, 1988).

Assessment of Functionally Related Variables

The mediating variables identified previously in the model of post-traumatic reactions among battered women are hypothesized to be functionally related as contributing causes (Brewer & Hunter, 1989) or as buffers in the development of such reactions. Another variable hypothesized to be functionally related consists of a battered woman's efforts to avoid, escape, or protect herself from the abuse. Thus, the assessment of these variables is an important component in comprehensive assessment, in addition to the assessment of PTSD and other symptoms per se.

EFFORTS AT AVOIDANCE, ESCAPE, OR PROTECTION FROM ABUSE

The assessment of battered women's efforts to avoid, escape, or protect themselves from abuse has relied primarily on interview procedures (Bowker, 1983; Gondolf with Fisher, 1988; Pagelow, 1981). Interviews can be open-ended, although structured interviews that present specific options may provide more complete data. A written questionnaire, the Response to Violence Inventory (Dutton, Hass, & Hohnecker, 1989), has been used within the Family Violence Program to assess (1) the frequency with which specific strategies have been used in the past; (2)

their perceived short-term effectiveness (i.e., their effectiveness in protecting a woman from abuse in the immediate situation); and (3) for specific strategies never employed (e.g., calling police), the rationale for not using them. The questionnaire is most useful when administered prior to a follow-up interview, which can provide an opportunity to elicit more detail. In addition, it is important to allow the battered woman the opportunity for spontaneous description of her unique and often amazingly creative efforts to protect herself, her children, and others from abuse.

OTHER CURRENT STRESSORS

Interview methods are useful for identifying specific sources of stress, in addition to the abuse, in the lives of battered women. Standard clinical tools used for measurement of current stress and the presence of existing stressors in the environment may prove useful. A comprehensive assessment must consider that the battered woman may be responding not only to the stress of previous and perhaps ongoing threats of abuse, but also to many other possible stressors (e.g., illness of child or parent, job stress), including those that may follow from the abuse (e.g., loss of home, children, income).

Secondary, or institutional, victimization (Stark & Flitcraft, 1989) must routinely be considered as a possible source of additional stress to the battered woman. Victim blaming or failure of law enforcement to provide protection, as well as lack of adequate assistance from a prosecutor, judge, medical professional, or psychotherapist, can compound the battered woman's level of stress resulting directly from the abuse alone.

SOCIAL SUPPORT AND OTHER RESOURCES

Interviews to assess the level of perceived social support to which the battered woman has access is important. It is useful to distinguish between perceived level of support and the availability of family or friends or even the extent of social contact. For some battered women, there is little social support available within their social network even though it may be quite extensive.

The Interpersonal Support Evaluation List (Cohen, Mermelstein, Kamarck, & Hoberman, 1985) has been used with battered women to distinguish the perceived availability of tangible resources, appraisal of support available, sense of belonging, and self-esteem. Data indicate that level of social support is related to level of distress among battered women (Dutton et al., 1990).

Education, occupational, and economic resources are also important variables that are hypothesized to mediate the development of post-traumatic stress reactions. At this time, these can best be evaluated through an interview method.

SUSCEPTIBILITY FACTORS

Historical factors that increase a battered woman's susceptibility to the traumatic effects of victimization must also be considered in the context of a comprehensive assessment. Relevant targets for assessment include (1) prior victimization (e.g., childhood sexual or physical abuse, rape, abuse in a prior adult relationship, sexual exploitation by professional, violence in childhood home) (Walker, 1984); (2) uncontrollable events in childhood (e.g., alcoholic parent, critical losses) (Walker, 1984); and (3) physical or mental disability, or any other historical factor that renders the battered woman as more vulnerable in the present context of an abusive relationship. Assessment conducted primarily through interview methods is recommended.

ASPECTS OF INTIMATE RELATIONSHIP OTHER THAN ABUSE

Not all aspects of a battered woman's relationship with her abusive partner may be experienced by the woman as negative. The occurrence of abuse may alternate with periods of time in which the relationship is experienced as relatively positive. The balance between positive and negative aspects (including those other than the abuse itself) of the intimate relationship is hypothesized to influence the development of PTSD and other psychological symptoms that result from intimate abuse. Although standard measures of relationship satisfaction may be of some use (e.g., the Dyadic Adjustment Scale; Spanier, 1976), interview methods may more adequately assess the specific situational determinants or the context under which the battered woman may experience the relationship as positive. For example, some women report that when their partners are not drinking they are pleasant and easy-going. On the other hand, in some battering relationships, the abuse is but one factor among several (e.g., infidelity) that contribute to dissatisfaction in the relationship.

PERSONALITY VARIABLES

Personality variables, including the three basic repertoires—language–cognitive, sensory–motor, and emotional–motivation (Staats, 1986) —are hypothesized to mediate the functional relationship between the experience of abuse and PTSD, as well as other psychological symptoms. Prior victimization may influence the development of personality (Herman, Perry, & van der Kolk, 1989), as may other life experiences. Rigid sex-role socialization (Walker, 1984) and low self-esteem or self-efficacy (Bandura, 1986) may provide the woman who is subsequently battered with few repertoires to respond effectively to the abuse against her. Assessment methods focused on specific targets are required. Although abuse may create PTSD and other symptoms in any woman, deficient personality repertoires may render the battered woman even more vulnerable.

Issues in Assessment

Several important issues should be considered in assessing PTSD and other psychological symptoms among battered women. These factors affect the outcome of assessment, as well as the assessment process itself.

DELAYED REACTION

Delayed PTSD is considered to occur when the onset of symptoms is at least 6 months after the event. For most battered women, the occurrence of trauma is not a discrete event with a clearly defined end point. Thus, identification of post-traumatic responses to trauma may be easily confused with the battered woman's traumatic responses (i.e., responses that occur during the course of the traumatic event), including those which she uses to attempt to protect herself from further abuse. For example, some battered woman use substances (e.g., alcohol, prescription or street drugs) in an attempt to manage their intense emotions. In such cases, a formal assessment may reveal very little evidence of classic PTSD intrusion or avoidance symptoms. The use of substances may be interpreted as a mechanism of avoidance, but there may be little indication of other avoidance symptoms as reported by the battered woman. When there is evidence of PTSD symptoms, the battered woman may not associate them with the occurrence of abuse. A comprehensive assessment of a battered woman's trauma-related symptoms must consider the influence of actual current threats of abuse as well as her use of alcohol and drugs, both of which may mask evidence of PTSD. Accurate assessment of PTSD may require waiting until the battered woman is in an environment where she feels at a safe distance from the threat of abuse (Horowitz, 1986).

IMPACT OF ASSESSMENT PROCEDURES

The process of participating in an assessment related to domestic abuse can be be stressful for a battered woman. Describing the nature and extent of abuse, recounting the extent of physical injuries, recognizing the psychological consequences of abuse, and identifying the extensive list of efforts she has made to protect herself (often without success) can quite vividly recreate the emotional climate of abuse for the battered woman. Sometimes the assessment experience may reconfirm a decision to leave the abusive relationship. Or the assessment may create such a vivid image of the abusive relationship that the battered woman cannot easily tolerate the reality of, it especially if she remains in that relationship. When a comprehensive assessment includes an accounting of prior victimization experiences (e.g., childhood abuse, prior rape) as well, the impact for the battered woman may be considerable.

It is important for trauma therapists to recognize that battered women's experiences include elements of both victimization and successful survival, in order to avoid two common pitfalls. The first, failing to identify the element of survival, increases the risk that the battered woman will continue to feel powerless and perhaps hopeless. The second, failing to recognize the battering experience as abuse or to acknowledge its impact, can leave the battered woman feeling psychologically invalidated. Thus, the process of assessment, like that of intervention, must include a close monitoring of the battered woman's responses to it.

Treatment

General Philosophy of Intervention with Battered Women

A core set of general assumptions has been proposed as necessary for working effectively with battered women (Dutton, in press). The following 13 assumptions have been adapted from Wilson (1989), Schechter (1987), and Courtois (1988), among others.

1.   Nonjudgemental acceptance and validation of a battered woman and her experiences are essential therapist goals. Blaming the battered woman for her abuse revictimizes her. However, nonjudgmental acceptance does not preclude examining behaviors of the battered woman that may have ineffectively protected the woman against the dangers of abuse, or that may be illegal or against her best interest.

2.   A therapist must be prepared to provide support, alliance, and advocacy for safety and building options. The therapist's support may be the only support available to the battered woman. Advocating for safety does not mean mandating any particular action by the battered woman.

3.   A therapists must be willing to be exposed to the recounting of the traumatic experience and its sequelae. The therapist must be skilled at listening and encouraging the battered woman to talk about details of her abusive experiences. Otherwise, these experiences remain inaccessible to effective intervention.

4.   It is assumed that PTSD and related symptoms are caused by the traumatic events, not by pre-existing personality factors. The traumatic experience of domestic abuse is considered necessary and sufficient to result in significant psychological symptoms, even though other factors may mediate or compound such reactions.

5.   Education is therapeutic. Education about typical post-traumatic reactions can "normalize" these responses for battered women. Furthermore, education about the prevelance of abuse within intimate relationships can enable the battered woman to understand her individual situation within the broader social context in which abuse occurs.

6.   Therapist self-care is essential. There is a risk of vicarious traumatization in being exposed to the abusive experiences described by battered women. Accordingly, therapists need to monitor their own reactions and maintain self-care in order to avoid long-term negative consequences for themselves and their clients.

7.   Coping strategies should be described as strengths, rather than being labeled as stable personality factors. Efforts to cope with the trauma of abuse and violence in an intimate relationship represent a strength, regardless of the effectiveness of those efforts in preventing further abuse.

8.   Self-medication or numbing is common among battered women. Although the use of drugs or alcohol undoubtedly has detrimental side effects, and substance abuse requires attention, its function in self-medicating against the experience of trauma needs to be recognized in order for effective intervention to occur.

9.   Transformation of the traumatic response may result in positive changes. The process of surviving, escaping, and transforming the trauma may lead to more than simply the removal of dysfunctional symptomatology. Recognition and development of personal coping skills, including an increased perception of self-efficacy or empowerment, may also result.

10.   Prosocial action and self-disclosure facilitate the stress recovery process. Engaging in overt behavior directed toward challenging the social problems associated with domestic abuse can create a sense of self-efficacy and empowerment over the abuse.

11.   Transformation of the trauma experienced by the battered woman may be a life-long process, even though specific symptoms may be alleviated at any given point in time. Events in a battered woman's lifetime, long after the original course of intervention is completed, may challenge her by triggering a recurrence of PTSD symptoms. These should be interpreted not as treatment failure, but as part of a normal course of recovery from trauma.

12.   Losses associated with abuse and victimization may be noncompensable, not able to be reclaimed; however, they can be grieved for. Even though a battered woman may remarry or regain financial stability, for example, she may never replace the losses she experiences. She may only recover from the psychological effects resulting from them.

13.   It is assumed that the battered woman has the right to self-determination; she is entitled to make her own decisions, regardless of whether they correspond with those of her therapist or others around her. Without the assumption of self-determination, the battered woman lives under the control of someone else. Even when the "someone else" professes benevolent intentions, this is not unlike the situation in which she finds herself with the abusive partner.

Interventions Related to Safety and Choice-Making Concerns

Clinical intervention with battered women can be organized around three basic concerns: (1) safety, (2) choice making, and (3) post-traumatic reactions. These concerns are applicable both to battered women still facing danger from their abusive partners and to those who have achieved some distance from danger.

Goals associated with concerns of safety include helping to protect a woman from further abuse and, where necessary, from the risk of suicidal or homicidal behaviors. In addition, support and protection during crises involving acute and intense emotional reactions, including brief psychotic reactions, may be necessary. These issues are relevant regardless of whether the battered woman is living in a relationship with her abuser or not. Although the principal focus of this chapter is on intervention with PTSD, attention must be paid also to interventions that focus on choice making. A brief discussion of interventions to address safety and choice-making concerns is necessary to provide a clinical context within which PTSD therapy with battered women can appropriately be considered.

PROVISION OF INFORMATION AND DEVELOPMENT OF PLANS

To address concerns of increasing protection against further abuse, the battered woman should always be provided with basic information about resources available in her community. These include information about battered women's shelters or safe houses; information about law enforcement's authority to make a domestic violence arrest under existing state law; information about the availability of injunctions for protection; procedures for obtaining one, and sanctions for violation; and information about the limits of an injunction's ability to protect an individual against physical force.

The development of escape and protection plans is also an important component of intervention toward the goal of safety. The need to articulate in detail an escape plan (a plan to escape or avoid abuse) or a protection plan (a plan for minimizing injury once abuse is inevitable and escape is not likely) can be introduced by the therapist. Although the primary goal is to increase the likelihood that the battered woman can escape or survive a subsequent episode of abuse, a secondary effect can be to increase her recognition of the level of danger that she faces. This recognition may lead her to place an even higher priority on intensifying efforts to maintain the safety of her children and herself. Thus, the therapist can rarely afford the luxury of assuming that safety is no longer an issue. A battered woman often lives in the shadow of the batterer's threat that he will someday find her, perhaps when she least expects it, and seriously injure or kill her. Any therapist working with battered women will inevitably also be required to attend to issues of safety.

"Choice making" as a goal refers to decision making and problem solving, usually related to such concerns as whether to leave or return to the abusive relationship, whether to move away from the abuser's community and/or to assume a different identity, whether to obtain a job or to change jobs, and how to provide for care of the children. These issues, like those of safety, are relevant for the battered woman regardless of the status of her relationship with the abuser.

Probably the most critical choice point for the battered woman is her decision to leave, stay in, or return to the abusive relationship. Many battered women seeking help for PTSD symptoms and related distress will also be facing this decision simultaneously. Specifically, the goal of intervention is to help a battered woman make a decision that reflects her own informed choice. Her right to decision making also means that she has a right to choose to remain in the relationship, regardless of the therapist's feelings about that. Some therapists have been known to refuse treatment if battered women do not choose to leave their abusive relationships. Such use of coercive power by a therapist clearly negates an assumption of self-determination on the part of the battered woman.

PROBLEM SOLVING: A TOOL FOR CHOICE MAKING

A problem-solving paradigm (D'Zurilla, 1986; Nezu & Nezu, 1989) provides a useful framework for working toward goals of choice making with the battered woman. The general process of problem solving involves the sequence of several steps: (1) identifying and describing the problem; (2) identifying and describing thoughts, feelings, and any other available information about the problem; (3) identifying alternative choices or responses to the problem, costs and benefits associated with each, and potential obstacles to each possible choice; (4) selecting a choice; (5) detailing a plan to implement the choice; (6) implementing the selected choice, including efforts toward countering barriers and obstacles to action; and (7) evaluating the choice concerning its effectiveness in solving the problem.

SPECIFIC TECHNIQUES

Within a problem-solving approach to choicemaking, the use of specific techniques may be incorporated, including education, support, skill development, development of strategies for reducing interference with routine functioning, and social and political activism to counter social barriers to the battered woman. Examples of specific goals using these techniques include the following.

1. Increasing self-nurturing behaviors may be necessary to reestablish battered women's sense of individuality, dignity, and personal worth, which are basic emotional needs. Thus, a focus on attending to residual physical injuries, nutrition, exercise, and rest may be important.

Identifying emotional needs and ways to get these needs met is one manner of increasing a battered woman's resources for engaging in choice making.

2. Increasing the battered woman's knowledge about abuse and its effects may facilitate her ability to make effective choices about leaving, staying in, or returning to an abusive relationship. Recognizing that her abusive situation is part of a larger social problem helps to create a different perspective from which she may respond. Education about common post-traumatic effects of abuse may also enable her to understand her own responses, which she may have failed to associate with her victimization.

3. Increasing the social and economic resources to which the battered woman has access increases the options from which she can choose. Information about social service resources within the community can create numerous options that are otherwise unavailable to the battered woman. Social support provided during times of crisis can also be a powerful buffer in reducing post-traumatic distress.

4. Challenging assumptions and cognitions about the violence is useful in overcoming the cognitive barriers to effective problem solving. Useful cognitive interventions include (a) reframing (e.g., the battered woman's response to psychological abuse can be reframed as a normal reaction to trauma; her perception of her situation can be reframed as including choices rather than as permitting no choice); (b) challenging minimization and denial of abuse or its psychological impact on the battered woman or her children; (c) reattributing responsibility for abuse to the one who initiates it, not to the one who uses physical force to defend against it; (d) attributing personal responsibility to the battered woman for her own safety and well-being; and (e) increasing perception of viable alternatives within available resources.

5. Challenging socialized sex-role beliefs may be necessary to overcome strong barriers to a battered woman's efforts to protect herself in an abusive situation. Helping a battered woman to examine her belief system, and the constraints that it places on her, may assist her in creating more options from which to respond to her victimization.

6. Increasing independent living skills may be important, since critical skill deficits in this area may prevent many battered women from leaving an abusive situation. A battered woman may have deficits in adequate income-producing skills, instrumental living skills (e.g., financial management, household or car maintenance), or social skills. Skill deficits may have resulted from a lack of opportunity in a sexist or racist society; thus, the deficits should not automatically be viewed as an indication of a battered woman's personal failure.

7. Increasing coping skills to deal with effects of victimization, as distinct from therapy to reduce or eliminate related psychological distress, may be necessary to help the battered woman reduce interference with her choice-making efforts. The development of coping skills may include strategies for the management of symptoms (e.g., depressed mood, anxiety, phobic reactions including agoraphobia, sleep and eating disturbances), rather than removal of the symptoms. Until control of the threat of continued abuse is achieved, it is not realistic to expect symptom removal to be achieved. Addressing the battered woman's use of harmful coping strategies (e.g., excessive alcohol and drug use, self-abuse, use of aggression toward children) may be necessary.

Interventions with PTSD Symptoms and Related Distress

Treatment focused upon the post-traumatic effects of abuse is most relevant when the battered woman has effectively escaped the abusive relationship. When the battered woman can shift her primary concern from that of protection against abuse, she is able to focus on her recovery from the effects of abuse. However, the battered woman who remains within the abusive relationship may also require therapeutic attention to the effects of abuse, to enable her effective escape from the abusive situation.

My colleagues' and my intervention strategy for trauma-related symptoms is formulated upon the guiding conceptual model presented earlier in this chapter (see Figure 4.1). In our model, the traumatic experience of violence and abuse in an intimate relationship is necessary and sufficient to produce the effects described as post-traumatic stress reactions. Attention is also given to intervention with the mediating factors that are hypothesized to be functionally related to the post-traumatic stress reaction. Effective intervention with battered women, as with other trauma victims, requires attention to the whole person (Ochberg, 1988).

Psychological treatment for PTSD has been described consistently as involving two phases: re-exposure to the trauma and management of related distress (Foa et al., 1989; Horowitz, 1986). In this chapter, PTSD treatment for battered women is discussed in the context of four therapeutic tasks that are viewed as important elements to promote trauma processing for the experience of being battered. In particular, increased attention is paid to cognitive and emotion-focused sequelae of traumatic victimization (Foa et al., 1989; McCann & Pearlman, 1990a). The four critical therapeutic tasks are these: (1) re-experiencing the traumatic events; (2) managing the subsequent stress; (3) facilitating expression of emotion, including shame, rage, and grief; and (4) finding meaning from the victimization. These therapeutic tasks should not be considered to be linear. They cannot be accomplished in clearly delineated stages, since each task may require attention at almost any point in the therapeutic process. Thus, the course of therapy should be modified according to the battered woman's individual needs.

RE-EXPERIENCING THE TRAUMA

Re-experiencing the trauma as a means of integrating the experience has been described as important across a variety of trauma groups (Courtois, 1988; Horowitz, 1986; McCann & Pearlman, 1990a; Steketee & Foa, 1987). The primary purpose of facilitating the battered woman's re-experiencing the traumatic abuse is reduction of both generalized fear and trauma-related intrusive thoughts, images, flashbacks, and nightmares. It is important to underscore that exposure to any stimuli that may actually present a threat may realistically and appropriately produce a strong emotional reaction; no attempt should be made to alter these reactions. The re-experiencing process is one that may require multiple exposures in order to achieve the goals described above. Both the level of avoidance and the intensity of intrusive experience prior to intervention may influence the extent to which re-experiencing is required.

Although systematic desensitization and flooding procedures, as methods of counterconditioning, have been used extensively with some trauma groups—for example, with Vietnam veterans (Keane, Fairbank, Caddell, & Zimering, 1989), and to some extent with rape trauma survivors (Frank & Stewart, 1983)—concerns have been expressed about the use of these methods (Courtois, 1988; Kilpatrick, Veronen, & Resick, 1982; McCann & Pearlman, 1990a). I suggest that those concerns apply to battered women as well. Specifically, the concern centers around the possibility of retraumatization, or repeated trauma, as a result of the too intense or too rapid re-exposure to the traumatic stimuli that may occur with flooding. Furthermore, re-experiencing trauma requires a trusting and supportive environment in which the battered woman can feel emotionally safe, in order for the experience to be a therapeutic rather than a retraumatizing one. For the battered woman, the therapeutic re-exposure will most likely occur in the context of retelling her story and other more naturalistic conditions. Thus, although general procedures for flooding or desensitization are not recommended for battered women, therapists cannot avoid reexposure altogether, nor should they. The fear memory must be activated in order to make it available for modification

(Foa et al., 1989). Of course, any intervention requires the informed and voluntary consent of the battered woman.

Integration of trauma through re-experiencing requires a here-and-now experience, rather than a detached reporting of events. Verbally recounting the abusive experiences in the therapy environment, however, may be sufficient to trigger the emotional component of re-experiencing the trauma. The therapist can use a variety of strategies to enable the battered woman to experience a greater or lesser amount of emotion associated with recounting abuse experiences. Moreover, the battered woman will self-regulate the amount of exposure by her willingness to respond to the therapist's cues for greater or lesser emotional experience. The re-experiencing process thus can proceed with varying degrees of exposure to trauma, paralleling the exposure component of systematic desensitization; however, it is more informal and less structured or hierarchical, and it is controlled to a greater extent by the client.

When avoidance of the traumatic memory is the predominant clinical presentation, strategies for intensification of emotion may be necessary. Such strategies include slowing down the process of recounting the experience to include greater detail, refocusing awareness on inner (i.e., affective/physiological, imaginal) experience, increasing the vividness of imagery, intensifying general level of arousal by increasing physical level of activity, physically enacting what is being described, and exaggerating or repeating phrases (Edwards, 1989; Greenberg & Safran, 1989). The use of photographs or documents describing the abuse may be useful in triggering the re-experience for the battered woman.

Facilitating a shift in cognitive fear structures related to traumatic experience (Foa et al., 1989) is a major component of this intervention. An essential element of working with fear structures is the modification of the current threat meaning of the conditioned stimuli associated with prior traumatization (e.g., sex with a new partner who has never been abusive, loud voices heard in the course of an argument with someone who poses no threat of violence, being alone in one's house). Cognitive fear structures can be modified by the habituation of arousal within sessions (Foa & Kozak, 1986); each time the battered woman recounts her experience in the emotionally safe environment of the therapy session, new information about the presence of fear is introduced. Furthermore, new information must be introduced to include components that are incompatible with some of those that exist in the fear structure so new memories can be formed. "This new information, which is at once cognitive and affective, has to be integrated into the evoked information structure for an emotional change to occur" (Foa & Kozak, 1986, p. 22). Helping the formerly battered woman integrate information about the probability of current harm from the conditioned stimuli is expected to reduce the intensity of the fear response. New affective and cognitive memories are formed when the battered woman's memories and images associated with prior abuse are accompanied by an awareness of her current physical, affective, and cognitive experience of safety. Thus, before interventions involving reexperiencing can be effective, a deliberate effort is required to create an environment (both inside and outside the therapy session) in which the battered woman experiences both physical and emotional safety.

Working toward integrating the trauma of domestic abuse through re-experiencing may trigger re-experiencing of previous traumatic experiences, such as childhood sexual or physical abuse, rape by a stranger or a previous partner, prior physical assault, or sexual exploitation by a professional. The therapist should be prepared to respond to the emergence of issues related to these prior victimization experiences. First, recognizing that clients' post-traumatic responses may constitute a complex array of emotions and behaviors related to different traumatic experiences is important. Second, prioritizing (or reprioritizing) interventions with multiple prior traumatic experiences is important in order to establish a systematic approach to treatment, while simultaneously recognizing that various traumatic experiences may not be neatly compartmentalized. Finally, tailoring post-traumatic therapy to the unique constellation of traumatic experiences for a particular client is imperative. Further development of interventions that take these issues into account is needed.

MANAGING STRESS

Sometimes it is important to deintensify emotion, rather than to increase it, when intrusion experiences are too overwhelming. During the course of treatment, when the intensity of re-experiencing the trauma is too great, excessive physiological arousal may interfere with the battered woman's attention to information that can provide her with new meaning structures (Foa et al., 1989). Alternatively, the battered woman may be experiencing intrusion symptoms spontaneously in the form of images, intrusive thoughts, flashbacks, and nightmares. Strategies for reducing intensity of arousal include (1) refocusing attention to the external reality, away from internal cognitive and affective/physiological processes; (2) teaching relaxation techniques; (3) teaching skills of "dosing"—that is, moving attention toward and away from traumatic experience (Courtois, 1988); (4) developing structure around time, activities, and information; (5) increasing personal rest and reduction of external demands; (6) teaching skills to discriminate present from prior abusive situations; and (7) providing support and helping the woman develop support outside the therapeutic relationship. These strategies can be taught to the battered woman to use outside as well as during the therapy session.

FACILITATING EXPRESSION OF EMOTION

Facilitating the identification and expression of emotion associated with trauma is encouraged during the process of re-experiencing. Expression rather than avoidance of feelings is the goal. Creating an emotionally safe environment is, of course, essential in order to facilitate both the re-experiencing of trauma and the expression of affect associated with it. Emotions commonly associated with trauma include fear/terror, anger/rage, shame, and grief. Expression may take many forms, including expression in spoken words, in a journal, through the use of sounds (i.e., screaming, crying, moaning), or through art or movement. Particular care should be taken to ensure that feelings are expressed in a manner that does not imperil the safety of either the battered woman or others around her. The woman may need to be encouraged to "dose" the re-experiencing of trauma both inside and outside the therapy session, in order to limit strong feelings and to be able to express them in an environment providing an adequate level of support.

It is important to consider the expression of emotions related to abuse as a process, not an event. Moreover, the formerly battered woman may experience seemingly different emotions simultaneously or within a short time period. For example, feelings of anger about being sexually abused by one's intimate partner may be followed closely by feelings of guilt or shame, which in turn may trigger feelings of loss or love for the partner. It is important that all feelings be accepted and validated by the therapist. Decisions about how to orchestrate the expression of these feelings can be discussed overtly with the client.

FINDING MEANING FROM VICTIMIZATION

Finding meaning from traumatic events is an essential cognitive component of post-traumatic therapy (Janoff-Bulman, 1985; McCann & Pearlman, 1990a; Peterson & Seligman, 1983; Veronen & Kilpatrick, 1983). It includes establishing a purpose of the abuse; re-establishing a sense of controllability and predictability in one's life; and rebuilding shattered assumptions or cognitive schemas about self, the world, and others (e.g., self-blame for abuse, hopelessness, belief that all men are abusive or that trust and intimacy in relationships is never safe, belief that self is worthless). Principles of cognitive therapies (Beck, 1976; Edwards, 1989; McMullin, 1986; Meichenbaum, 1977; Muran & DiGiuseppe, 1990; Veronen & Kilpatrick, 1983) can be used to modify these beliefs, attributions, and appraisals. Most importantly, finding meaning and modifying belief systems can occur most effectively in coordination with re-experiencing the trauma and expressing of feelings, not as a process separate from these.

For example, one battered woman came to believe that her experience of physical, sexual, and psychological victimization by an intimate partner resulted in her becoming aware of what she termed the "realities" of the world—experiences about which she had previously had little awareness. She further believed that she now must learn to accept a "dark" side of herself, the part that felt anger and hate. This new view provided a purpose that had been gained from her torturous experiences.

Issues in Treatment with Battered Women

Several general issues in treatment with battered women that are important to consider include the following: (1) the social context of treatment, (2) the risk of retraumatization, (3) diversity issues, and (4) issues that affect the therapist.

SOCIAL CONTEXT OF TREATMENT

Effective assessment and treatment of post-traumatic stress reactions in battered women requires consideration of the functional analysis of the broad social context in which violence and abuse directed toward women occurs. Failing to account for components of the social environment that support abuse of women leaves the assessment of traumatic effects of domestic abuse at the dyadic, or worse, the individual level of analysis. Furthermore, effective intervention requires attention to the social and environmental variables that are functionally related to the development and maintenance of post-traumatic stress reactions in battered women.

RISK OF RETRAUMATIZATION

The ineffective use of assessment and intervention methods can retraumatize battered women. The use of controlling and rigid behavior by the therapist can risk exposing the battered woman to a relationship characterized by exposure to trauma-inducing stimuli—in other words, a relationship that is similar to her formerly abusive and overcontrolled relationship with the batterer. As mentioned earlier, particular clinical methods themselves (e.g., flooding) may risk retraumatizing battered women by virtue of the nature of the procedures. Above all else, the therapist should guard against the use of any assessment or intervention methods that place a battered woman at risk for retraumatization.

DIVERSITY ISSUES

Attention to the role of diversity issues (e.g., gender, race, class, sexual preference) is important in any attempt to understand the trauma of domestic abuse. Without the recognition that a poor, black battered woman may face quite a different response from the legal system in her efforts to protect herself from abuse than an upper-middle-class white woman might, for example, one may fail to account for the additional stress, scarcity of resources, and other factors that may affect the first woman's development and recovery from post-traumatic stress reactions. Recognition of how diversity issues between the therapist and client may affect the course of treatment is also important in guarding against the risk of revictimization—a risk that exists in a therapeutic relationship characterized by a large discrepancy in social power between therapist and client (Douglas, 1985).

The gender of the therapist is an important consideration in working with battered women. Certainly, any preference by the client for a therapist of either gender should be seriously considered. Some would argue that only women therapists should work with battered women. However, women therapists are not immune from beliefs and attitudes that can be detrimental to working with battered women. Furthermore, male therapists will encounter battered women and other female victims of violence, simply because of the vast number of victims who enter the mental health system. I believe that the most useful focus is on training both male and female therapists to work effectively with female victims of violence.

THERAPIST ISSUES

Recognition of the risk of vicarious traumatization (McCann & Pearlman, 1990b) is important if the therapists are to maintain their own well-being, as well as effective therapeutic skills with clients. Vicarious traumatization can negatively affect therapists' beliefs, attitudes, and emotions. Ochberg (1988) has stated:

Our work calls on us to confront, with our patients and within ourselves, extraordinary human experiences. This confrontation is profoundly humbling in that at all times these experiences challenge the limits of our humanity and our view of the world we live in. No matter how overwhelmingly tragic and painful, or how shocking and shameful, comprehending and integrating victimization are ultimately solidly grounding and thereby liberating both for our patients and for ourselves. (p. 293)

There is probably no professional experience more demanding than that of working with survivors of violence. A therapist must focus simultaneously on the battered woman and her needs, and on his or her own reactions and responses to working in that situation as a therapist.

Attention to personal attitudes, values, and needs holds a priority in working with survivors of violence and abuse that is unsurpassed in other forms of psychotherapy. A therapist needs to remain aware of the impact of his or her own victimization history, as well as of his or her vicarious traumatization experiences, in working with battered women. Supervision, peer support groups, attention to self-nurturing behaviors, diversification of professional activities so that not all of one's work is in direct clinical contact with survivors, and political activism against interpersonal violence may be effective as interventions for the therapist.

References

American Psychiatric Association. (1987). *Diagnostic and statistical manual of mental disorders* (3rd ed., rev.). Washington, D C: Author.

Bandura, A. (1986). *Social foundations of thought and action: A social cognitive theory.* Englewood Cliffs, NJ: Prentice-Hall.

Beck, A. T. (1976). *Cognitive therapy and the emotional disorders.* New York: New American Library.

Becker, R. E., & Heimberg, R. G. (1988). Assessment of social skills. In A. S. Bellack & M. Hersen (Eds.), *Behavioral assessment: A practical handbook* (3rd ed., pp. 365–395). Elmsford, NY: Pergamon Press.

Blackman, J. (1989). *Intimate violence: A study of injustice.* New York: Columbia University Press.

Bowker, L. H. (1983). *Beating wife-beating.* Lexington, MA: Lexington Books.

Brewer, J., & Hunter, A. (1989). *Multimethod research: A synthesis of styles.* Newbury Park, CA: Sage.

Browne, A. (1987). *When battered women kill.* New York: Free Press.

Campbell, J. (1989). A test of two explanatory models of women's responses to battering. *Nursing Research, 38*(1), 18–24.

Cimino, J. (1991). *Identification of post-traumatic stress disorder using the Crime-Related Post-Traumatic Stress Disorder Scale.* Unpublished manuscript, Nova University.

Cohen, S., Mermelstein, R., Kamarck, T., & Hoberman, H. N. (1985). Measuring the functional components of social support. In I. Sarason & B. Sarason (Eds.), *Social support: Theory, research, and applications* (pp. 73–94). Dordrecht, The Netherlands: Martinus Nijhoff.

Courtois, C. A. (1988). *Healing the incest wound: Adult survivors in therapy.* New York: Norton.

Douglas, M. A. (1985). The role of power in feminist therapy. In L. B. Rosewater & L. E. A. Walker (Eds.), *Handbook of feminist therapy: Women's issues in psychotherapy* (pp. 241–249). New York: Springer.

Douglas, M. A. (1987). Battered woman syndrome. In D. J. Sonkin (Ed.), *Domestic violence on trial* (pp. 39–54). New York: Springer.

Dutton, D., & Painter, S. L. (1981). Traumatic bonding: The development of emotional attachments in battered women and other relationships of intermittent abuse. *Victimology, 6,* 139–155.

Dutton, M. A. (in press). *Empowering and healing the battered woman: Assessment and treatment.* New York: Springer.

Dutton, M. A., Freeman, M. A., & Stumpff, A. (1988). *Abusive Behavior Observation Checklist.* Unpublished manuscript, Nova University.

Dutton, M. A., Hass, G., & Hohnecker, L. (1989). *Response to Violence Inventory.* Unpublished manuscript, Nova University.

Dutton, M. A., Perrin, S. G., Chrestman, K. R., & Halle, P. M. (1990, August). *MMPI trauma profiles for battered women.* Paper presented at the 98th Annual Convention of the American Psychological Association, Boston.

Dutton, M. A., Perrin, S. G., Chrestman, K. R., & Halle, P. M. (1991). *Concurrent validity of PTSD measures among battered women.* Manuscript submitted for publication.

Dutton-Douglas, M. A., Perrin, S., Chrestman, K. R. & Faden-Strauss, R. (1989, January). *Post-traumatic stress disorder: Battered women.* Paper presented at the Response to Family Violence Conference, Lafayette, IN.

D'Zurilla, T. J. (1986). *Problem solving therapy: A social competence approach to clinical intervention.* New York: Springer.

Edwards, D. J. (1989). Cognitive restructuring through guided imagery. In A. Freeman, K. M. Simon, L. E. Beutler, & H. Arkowitz (Eds.), *Comprehensive handbook of cognitive therapy* (pp. 283–297). New York: Plenum Press.

Fairbank, J. A. (1989). Chronic combat-related post-traumatic stress disorder. In A. M. Nezu & C. M. Nezu (Eds.), *Clinical decision-making in behavior therapy: A problem-solving perspective* (pp. 297–319). Champaign, IL: Research Press.

Foa, E. B., & Kozak, M. J. (1986). Emotional processing of fear: Exposure to corrective information. *Psychological Bulletin, 99,* 20–35.

Foa, E. B., Steketee, G., & Rothbaum, B. O. (1989). Behavioral/cognitive conceptualizations of post-traumatic stress disorder. *Behavior Therapy, 20,* 155–176.

Foy, D. W., Osato, S. S., Houskamp, B. M., & Neumann, D. A. (in press). PTSD etiology. In P. A. Saigh (Ed.), *Posttraumatic stress disorder: Behavioral assessment and treatment.* Elmsford, NY: Maxwell Press.

Foy, D. W., Rychtarik, R. G., & Prue, D. M (1988). Assessment of appetitive disorders. In A. S. Bellack & M. Hersen (Eds.), *Behavioral assessment: A practical handbook* (3rd ed. pp. 542–577). Elmsford, NY: Pergamon Press.

Frank, E., & Stewart, D. B. (1983). Treating depression in rape victims: A revisit. *Journal of Affective Disorders, 7*, 77–85.

Ganley, A. (Chair). (1981). *Court-mandated counseling for men who batter: A three-day workshop for mental health professionals.* Washington, DC: Center for Women's Policy Studies.

Ganley, A. (1989). Integrating feminist and social learning analyses of aggression: Creating multiple models for intervention with men who batter. In P. L. Caesar & L. K. Hamberger (Eds.), *Treating men who batter: Theory, practice, and programs* (pp. 196–235). New York: Springer.

Gondolf, E. W., with Fisher, E. R. (1988). *Battered women as survivors: An alternative to treating learned helplessness.* Lexington, MA: Lexington Books.

Graham, D. L. R., Rawlings, E., & Rimini, N. (1988). Survivors of terror: Battered women, hostages, and the Stockholm syndrome. In K. Yllo & M. Bograd (Eds.), *Feminist perspectives on wife abuse* (pp. 217–233). Beverly Hills, CA: Sage.

Greenberg, L. S., & Safran, J. D. (1989). Emotion in psychotherapy. *American Psychologist, 44*(1), 19–29.

Haynes, S. N., & O'Brien, W. H. (1990). Functional analysis in behavior therapy. *Clinical Psychology Review, 10*, 649–668.

Herman, J. D., Perry, J. C., & van der Kolk, B. A. (1989). Childhood trauma in borderline personality disorder. *American Journal of Psychiatry, 146*(4), 490–495.

Hilberman, E., & Munson, K. (1978). Sixty battered women. *Victimology, 2*, 460–470.

Horowitz, M. J. (1986). *Stress response syndromes* (2nd ed.). Northvale, NJ: Jason Aronson.

Horowitz, M. J., Wilner, N., & Alvarez, W. (1979). Impact of Event Scale: A measure of subjective stress. *Psychosomatic Medicine, 41*(3), 209–218.

Houskamp, B. M., Foy, D. W., & Baranoff, E. C. (1989, October). *The assessment of post-traumatic stress disorder in battered women.* Paper presented at the convention of the International Society for Traumatic Stress Studies, San Francisco.

Janoff-Bulman, R. (1985). The aftermath of victimization: Rebuilding shattered assumptions. In C. R. Figley (Ed.), *Trauma and its wake: Vol. 1. The study and treatment of post-traumatic stress disorder* (pp. 15–35). New York: Brunner/Mazel.

Janoff-Bulman, R., & Frieze, I. H. (1983). A theoretical perspective for understanding reactions to victimiztions. *Jouranl of Social Issues, 39*(2), 1–17.

Jaffee, P., Wolfe, D. A., Wilson, S., & Zak, L. (1986). Emotional and physical health problems of battered women. *Canadian Journal of Psychiatry, 31*(7), 625–629.

Keane, T. M. Fairbank, J. A., Caddell, J. A., & Zimering, R. T. (1989). Implosive (flooding) therapy reduces symptoms of PTSD in Vietnam combat veterans. *Behavior Therapy, 20*, 245–260.

Keane, T. M., Malloy, P. F., & Fairbank, J. A. (1984). Empirical development of an MMPI subscale for the assessment of combat related post–traumatic stress disorder. *Journal of Consulting and Clinical Psychology, 52*, 888–891.

Kilpatrick, D. G., Veronen, L. J., & Resick, P. A. (1982). Psychological sequelae to rape: Assessment and treatment strategies. In D. M. Doleys, R. L. Meredith, & A. R. Ciminero (Eds.), *Behavioral medicine: Assessment and treatment strategies* (pp. 473–497). New York: Plenum Press.

Koss, J. P., Woodruff, W. J., & Koss, P. G. (1990). Relation of criminal victimization to health perceptions among women medical patients. *Journal of Consulting and Clinical Psychology, 58*(2), 147–152.

McCann, I. L., & Pearlman, L. A. (1990a). *Psychological trauma and the adult survivor: Theory, therapy, and transformation.* New York: Brunner/Mazel.

McCann, I. L., & Pearlman, L. A. (1990b). Vicarious traumatization: A framework for understanding the psychological effects of working with victims. *Journal of Traumatic Stress, 3*(1), 131–149.

McCann, I. L., Sakheim, D. K., & Abrahamson, D. J. (1988). Trauma and victimization: A model of psychological adaptation. *The Counseling Psychologist, 16*(4), 531–594.

McMullin, R. E. (1986). *Handbook of cognitive therapy techniques.* New York: Norton.

Meichenbaum, D. (1977). *Cognitive-behavior modification: An integrative approach.* New York: Plenum Press.

Muran, I. C., & DiGiuseppe, R. A. (1990). Toward a cognitive formulation of metaphor use in psychotherapy. *Clinical Psychology Review, 10,* 69–85.

Neitzel, M. T., Bernstein, D. A., & Russell, R. L. (1988). Assessment of anxiety and fear. In A. S. Bellack & M. Hersen (Eds.), *Behavioral assessment: A practical handbook* (3rd ed., pp. 279–312). Elmsford, NY: Pergamon Press.

Nezu, A. M., & Nezu, C. M. (Eds.). (1989). *Clinical decision-making in behavior therapy: A problem-solving perspective.* Champaign, IL: Research Press.

Novaco, R. W. (1979). The cognitive regulation of anger and stress. In P. C. Kendall & S. D. Hollon (Eds.), *Cognitive–behavioral interventions: Theory, research and procedures.* New York: Academic Press.

Ochberg, F. M. (1988). Post–traumatic therapy and victims of violence. In F. M. Ochberg (Ed.), *Post-traumatic therapy and victims of violence* (pp. 3–19). New York: Brunner/Mazel.

Pagelow, M. D. (1981). *Woman-battering: Victims and their experiences.* Beverly Hills, CA: Sage.

Pence, E. (1987). *In our best interest.* Duluth: Minnesota Program Development.

Pence, E., & Paymar, M. (1986). *Power and control: Tactics of men who batter.* Duluth: Minnesota Program Development.

Peterson, C., & Seligman, M. (1988). Learned helplessness and victimization. *Journal of Social Issues, 2,* 103–116.

Rehm, L. P. (1988). Assessment of depression. In A. S. Bellack & M. Hersen (Eds.), *Behavioral assessment: A practical handbook* (3rd ed., pp. 313–364). Elmsford, NY: Pergamon Press.

Rosal, M., Dutton-Douglas, M.A., & Perrin, S. (1990, August). *Anxiety in battered women.* Paper presented at the 98th Annual Convention of the American Psychological Association, Boston.

Saunders, B. E., Arata, C. M., & Kilpatrick, D. G. (1990). Development of a crime-related post-traumatic stress disorder scale for women within the Symptom Checklist-90-Revised. *Journal of Traumatic Stress, 3*(3), 439–448.

Saunders, D. G. (1990, June). *The traumatic aftermath of violence against women.* Paper presented at the Research Scientist Development Awardees Conference, Chevy Chase, MD.

Schechter, S. (1987). *Guidelines for mental health practitioners in domestic violence cases.* Washington, DC: National Coalition Against Domestic Violence.

Scrignar, C. B. (1988). *Post-traumatic stress disorder: Diagnosis, treatment, and legal issues* (2nd ed.). New Orleans: Bruno Press.

Spanier, G. B. (1976). Measuring dyadic adjustment: New scales for assessing the quality of marriage and similar dyads. *Journal of Marriage and the Family, 38,* 15–28.

Spitzer, R. L., & Williams, J. B. W. (1986). *Structured clinical interview for DSM-III-R.* New York: New York State Psychiatric Institute.

Staats, A. W. (1986). Behaviorism with a personality: The paradigmatic behavioral assessment approach. In R. O. Nelson & S. C. Hayes (Eds.), *Conceptual foundations of behavioral assessment* (pp. 242–295). New York: Guilford Press.

Stark, E., & Flitcraft, A. (1989). Personal power and institutional victimization: Treating the dual trauma of woman battering. In F. M. Ochberg (Ed.), *Post-traumatic therapy and victims of violence* (pp. 115–151). New York: Brunner/Mazel.

Stark, E., Flitcraft, A., Zuckerman, D., Grey, A., Robison, J., & Frazier, W. (1981). *Wife abuse in the medical setting: An introduction for health personnel.* Rockville, MD: National Clearinghouse on Domestic Violence.

Steketee, G., & Foa, E. B. (1987). Rape victims: Post-traumatic stress responses and their treatment: A review of the literature. *Journal of Anxiety Disorders, 1,* 69–86.

Straus, M. A. (1979). Measuring intrafamily conflict and violence: The Conflict Tactics (CT) Scales. *Journal of Marriage and the Family, 41,* 75–81.

Tolman, R. M. (1989). The development of a measure of psychological maltreatment of women by their male partners. *Violence and Victims, 4*(3), 159–177.

Trimpey, M. L. (1989). Self-esteem and anxiety: Key issues in an abused women's support group. Special issues: Family violence. *Issues in Mental Health Nursing, 10*(3–4), 297–308.

Turner, S. F., & Shapiro, C. H. (1986). Battered women: Mourning the death of a relationship. *Social Work, 31*(5), 372–376.

Veronen, L. J., & Kilpatrick, D. G. (1983). Stress management for rape victims. In D. Meichenbaum & M. Jaremko (Eds.), *Stress reduction and prevention* (pp. 341–374). New York: Plenum Press.

Walker, L. E. (1984). *Battered woman syndrome.* New York: Springer.

Watson, C. G. (1990). Psychometric post-traumatic stress disorder measurement techniques: A review. *Psychological Assessment, 2*(4), 460–469.

Williamson, D. A., Davis, C. J., & Prather, R. C. (1988). Assessment of health-related disorders. In A. S. Bellack & M. Hersen (Eds.), *Behavioral assessment: A practical handbook* (3rd ed., pp. 396–440). Elmsford, NY: Pergamon Press.

Wilson, J. P. (1989). *Trauma, transformation, and healing: An integrative approach to theory, research, and posttraumatic therapy.* New York: Brunner/Mazel.

5

Assessment and Treatment of Post-Traumatic Stress Disorder in Adult Survivors of Sexual Assault

HEIDI S. RESNICK and TAMARA NEWTON

The goal of this chapter is to describe assessment and treatment of adults with sexual-assault-related PTSD, as conducted at an outpatient trauma clinic, the Crime Victims Research and Treatment Center. Our discussion of assessment includes descriptions of the two major domains: (1) assessment of trauma characteristics; and (2) assessment of PTSD symptomatology using multiple methods. Our treatment approach, combining elements of skills training and exposure techniques, is then presented. Both of these behavioral strategies have been employed to treat PTSD related to sexual assault, and preliminary findings from treatment outcome studies support the efficacy of these techniques, relative to no-treatment control conditions.

Significance of the Problem

Sexual assault is currently included in the DSM-III-R as a type of traumatic stressor capable of precipitating the full pattern of PTSD symptoms. Thus, information about the prevalence of sexual assault, both in the general population and in clinical samples, is important. It provides a probability estimate for clients' exposure to a traumatic sexual assault and related risk for development of PTSD symptoms.

Sexual assault occurs frequently in the histories of women in both nonclinical and clinical populations. Less is known about prevalence in the male population. Results of epidemiological studies of nonclinical populations indicate that between one-fourth and one-half of women surveyed had experienced some form of sexual assault (Kilpatrick, Saunders, Veronen, Best, & Von, 1987; Kilpatrick & Best, 1990; Koss, Gidycz, & Wisniewski, 1987). Finally, a molestation rate of 13.2% was observed in a community sample of both males and females (Burnam et al., 1988). Thus, in general population samples, the base rate of sexual assault is high.

Higher rates of sexual assault have been observed in some clinical samples. Observed lifetime rates of sexual assault in outpatient and inpatient samples that included males and females have ranged from 20% to 50% (Saunders, Kilpatrick, Resnick, & Tidwell, 1989; Jacobson & Richardson, 1987). Finally, histories of childhood sexual abuse have been observed in approximately 50% of samples of female inpatients (Bryer, Nelson, Miller, & Krol, 1987; Beck & van der Kolk, 1987).

These findings establish the significance of sexual assault as a frequently occurring traumatic event. The second factor in further establishing the clinical relevance of the problem is the question of the likelihood that those exposed to sexual assault will develop PTSD. The results of studies conducted prior to the introduction of the PTSD diagnostic category indicated that rape and sexual assault survivors displayed clinically significant levels of anxiety and depressive symptoms (Atkeson, Calhoun, Resick, & Ellis, 1982; Kilpatrick, Veronen, & Resick, 1979; Frank, Turner, & Duffy, 1979).

More recent studies using PTSD diagnostic criteria show that the disorder occurs frequently following sexual assault. Kilpatrick, Saunders, et al. (1987) observed lifetime rates of PTSD ranging between 11.1% in association with attempted molestation and 57.1% in association with completed rape. One-third of the women with histories of completed molestation also developed PTSD. Results indicated that sexual-assault-related PTSD was chronic in many cases. A higher rate of PTSD has been observed in a longitudinal study of a sample referred by a crisis agency restricted to rape survivors only. Rothbaum, Foa, Riggs, Murdock, and Walsh (in press) found that 94% of this sample met criteria for PTSD at approximately 2 weeks after the rape, whereas approximately half of the group displayed PTSD at 12 weeks after the rape.

The data reviewed in this section have important clinical implications. First, sexual assault appears to be so common in clinical populations that routine screening for sexual assault history should be conducted with all female clients presenting for treatment (Kilpatrick, 1983). Second, the data support the applicability of a PTSD model in describing reactions to sexual assault. Thus, clients with an identified history of sexual assault should also receive routine assessment for PTSD.

Theoretical Models of Sexual-Assault-Related PTSD

Several cognitive–behavioral theories of PTSD development or maintenance have influenced the evolution of our methods for both assessment and treatment of sexual-assault-related PTSD. In one of the earliest formulations, Kilpatrick et al., (1979) proposed that two-factor learning theory was useful for conceptualizing postassault reactions. Principles of both classical and operant conditioning were proposed as central to the development and persistence of fear to cues associated with sexual assault trauma. It was also proposed that additional learning principles of stimulus generalization and higher-order conditioning lead to perpetuation of anxiety reactions to a broader array of stimuli.

More recently proposed models have focused more heavily on information processing and cognitive variables, such as perceived threat, predictability, and controllability, as central to development and/or maintenance of PTSD (Foa, Steketee, & Rothbaum, 1989; Jones & Barlow, 1990). In addition to stressing the importance of cognitive perception, these models place heavier emphasis on response elements as cues in a fear memory network that may elicit re-experiencing of symptoms (e.g., repetitive thoughts, memories, dreams, and alarm reactions). Other cognitive models stress the importance of the survivor's more global attributions about causality and appraisal of meaning in relation to sexual assault as affecting outcome (Veronen & Kilpatrick, 1983; Janoff-Bulman, 1985).

Finally, Jones and Barlow (1990) and Foy, Osato, Houskamp, and Neumann (in press) have proposed comprehensive mediational models that posit interactions between individual and stressor characteristics in the development and maintenance of PTSD. Both of these models suggest that variables such as social support, coping, family history, and past history of psychopathology may serve as either predisposing or protective factors in determining outcome following exposure to a potentially traumatic stressor. The models differ, however, in terms of the stage at which these variables are hypothesized as having a major impact. Although they recognize the important role of exposure characteristics, Jones and Barlow (1990) suggest that these mediational variables may determine initial reactions to trauma. In contrast, Foy et al. (in press) propose that stressor characteristics are necessary and sufficient for eliciting an acute reaction, whereas mediational variables may play a greater role in determining whether symptoms resolve or become chronic.

These behavioral models of PTSD development have provided the basis for our assessment and treatment strategies. In terms of assessment, the models described here suggest the importance of gathering information about (1) exposure characteristics of the trauma; (2) initial reactions to and cognitive perceptions about the traumatic experience; (3) stimulus and response components that have become part of a fear memory or signal for danger; and (4) psychosocial characteristics that may be associated with differential likelihood of PTSD development and maintenance. In terms of treatment, the models suggest the importance of therapeutic exposure to elements of the stimulus–response complex, to allow for reduction in anxiety and to facilitate dissociations between stimuli and responses. In addition, cognitive therapy aimed at facilitating accurate and adaptive interpretations of trauma is suggested. Information-processing models suggest that therapeutic exposure produces alterations in the cognitive perception of danger or other maladaptive interpretations associated with stimulus and response elements, and thus leads to reduction in PTSD symptoms (Foa et al., 1989; Foa & Kozak, 1986; Jones & Barlow, 1990).

Assessment

It is helpful to conceptualize the assessment of sexual-assault-related PTSD as targeting two broad areas: stressor and symptom characteristics. The stressor domain refers to the traumatic event and its characteristics, as described by the client and any supporting documentation (e.g., police reports). The symptom domain refers to the psychological sequelae of exposure to the stressor, as determined through client self-report, data from structured clinical interviews, laboratory data on psychophysiological responding and behavioral avoidance, and the clinician's observations regarding the client's functioning.

Generally, our assessment is conducted over the course of at least two sessions. At the initial meeting, emergent issues are addressed; in addition, we gather important psychosocial history information. In the stressor domain, we determine the type of sexual assault that has been experienced, as well as the presence of important trauma-related variables. To assess symptoms, we ask clients to describe presenting problems in an open-ended fashion, and also to complete a series of self-report instruments. Typically in the second session, we gather information about the entire lifetime history of traumatic events. In addition, we conduct a structured interview assessment of PTSD and any comorbid conditions indicated as presenting problems. Taken together, these components guide the identification of target symptoms and the development of a treatment plan for cases of sexual-assault-related PTSD. The following sections cover these basic components of assessment.

Assessment of Emergent Issues

Because the setting in which we see clients is an outpatient trauma clinic, it is important for us to assess emergent safety issues that may require immediate intervention and networking with other community agencies. In some cases, clients are in danger of being assaulted or have a pressing need for information about the legal system. In other cases, hospitalization may be required.

SUICIDALITY

At initial assessment it is important to assess whether clients might harm or attempt to kill themselves. The typical questions addressing this issue include asking whether clients are thinking about death, suicide, or self-harm. If responses are positive, they are followed up with questions about actual intent, available means, and any potential restraining factors (e.g., religious beliefs, relationships with significant others), as well as assessment of the seriousness and nature of any past attempts, and the client's ability to control their behavior and contract not to harm themselves. If a therapist believes that a client is at immediate risk for self-destructive behavior, then at least a brief hospital stay is recommended for additional evaluation of presenting problems. Often, the client recognizes the advisability of hospitalization under these circumstances. However, in a case where there is a serious threat of suicide, and no commitment can be obtained from the client to refrain from self-destructive behavior and hospitalization is refused, the therapist may have to take action to hospitalize the client involuntarily. In our setting, this requires an evaluation by a physician. In these rare instances, we call upon a mobile unit from the emergency room to make this evaluation.

POTENTIAL FOR VIOLENCE TOWARD OTHERS

Common reactions following sexual assault include fear of revictimization by the perpetrator and intense anger toward the perpetrator. It is important to assess the client's potential for retribution or for engaging in extreme behavior to prevent future attacks. A client who is having thoughts about harming the perpetrator will often spontaneously disclose this to the therapist. In other cases, a useful way to raise the subject is to find out what efforts have been made for self-protection, if any, since the assault. In some cases this will lead to disclosure of bearing weapons or having easy access to lethal weapons.

As in the case of suicidality, thoughts, intentions, likelihood of future interactions or confrontations with the perpetrator, and ability and willingness to use more constructive means for protection from future harm and seeking redress are assessed. If the therapist believes that someone is in serious danger of harm, he or she has an obligation to warn that person of this circumstance. In our experience, in the rare case in which this issue arises, we have been able to reach some agreement with the client that averts the necessity of warning the perpetrator. This has occasionally included an agreement by the client to relinquish a weapon to someone else who can be contacted by the therapist.

In many recent sexual assault cases, there is ongoing contact with the legal system, which can perpetuate the trauma or at least serve as a frequent reminder of the sexual assault. In addition, in a case in which the perpetrator has not been apprehended or has been released on bond, a client may have extreme fear of revictimization. During the initial assessment meeting, it is important to find out about the status of the legal process. If the client is deliberating about whether or not to press charges, it is important to clarify options available and potential consequences of actions taken. Although we may encourage clients to take legal action, our overriding goal is to help them make decisions for themselves. Often clients are unaware of community agencies that provide legal information and support. These include the local rape crisis center, which provides victim accompaniment at all stages of the legal process as well as liaison with the police. The police departments and prosecutors' offices also have special victim assistance agents who provide information and assistance. Our treatment center maintains links with these agencies, and we provide our clients with information about the services available to them.

Psychosocial History Variables That May Mediate Outcome

The role of individual or historical characteristics, such as past history of psychopathology, history of psychological or psychiatric treatment, family history of psychopathology, prior victimization, coping capabilities, and social support, has yet to be thoroughly investigated in the development or maintenance of assault-related PTSD. Findings remain unclear because most studies have not examined PTSD as an outcome variable, or have failed to control for the presence of differing assault characteristics, which may in themselves increase the risk of PTSD development.

However, since in our current behavioral conceptual model of PTSD these variables may affect either initial or longer-term reactions to trauma, they are important to assess. Pretrauma strengths or vulnerability factors may also help to guide treatment approaches. For example, successful coping techniques that an individual has used to deal with past stressors may be successfully employed in treatment. Conversely, maladaptive strategies that have become well ingrained may have to be specifically targeted in treatment. In addition, potential vulnerability factors, such as past history of psychopathology, may influence the development of PTSD symptoms or other disorders; this may well require a broadening of the scope of treatment.

At our initial assessment, we gather standard psychosocial history information. Areas covered include past history of psychiatric disorder, family history, past treatment seeking or hospitalization, past and current medication use, and history of serious physical illness. We also ask about social support available to the client and the responses of significant others to the assault. Asking about the client's daily routine, as well as basic demographic information, provides helpful information about current functioning. Finally, it is useful to find out about techniques the client is currently using to cope with anxiety. These may include either adaptive techniques (such as talking with others) or maladaptive strategies (such as increased substance use).

Assessment of the Trauma

Assessment of the traumatic history is conducted in the following order in our clinic. First, we identify the type of sexual assault experienced. Second, we identify potentially important trauma-related variables, including exposure and cognitive appraisal characteristics. Third, we conduct a routine assessment for other traumatic experiences in the client's history. Prior to discussing the trauma assessment measures that we use, we address potential barriers to clients' disclosure of their sexual assault and clinical approaches to overcome these barriers.

CLINICAL APPROACHES TO ELICIT DISCLOSURE

Importantly, we recognize potential barriers that may impede disclosure of sexual assault. Major client variables that may prevent disclosure include fear of being judged or blamed for the victimization; lack of awareness that sexual assault may be associated with presenting psychological or behavioral problems; and failure to identify objective incidents of abuse as sexual assault because they do not fit cultural stereotypes of what a sexual assault is like (Kilpatrick, 1983). It may also be that difficulties with disclosure can relate to cognitive or behavioral avoidance of the traumatic event.

Therapist variables that may impede routine assessment of sexual assault history include lack of knowledge of the high prevalence of sexual assault and its significance as a potential precipitant of PTSD. In addition, discomfort about using sexual terms and fear of upsetting clients may be inhibiting factors. Therapists should examine their own feelings and evaluate whether they are avoiding this important assessment to spare themselves discomfort or embarrassment. If so, they can desensitize themselves by becoming more familiar with terms and phrases included in the measures described below.

Regarding the fear of upsetting clients, it is more likely that ignoring this important history variable will result in harm or lack of benefit to the patients. In fact, it is often the case that clients may not have been supported in previous attempts at disclosure, or that the abuse may have been ignored by significant others. It is important that these negative responses are not repeated and that therapists empathically offer the opportunity for disclosure. A therapist should consider the possible negative messages to a client that may result from displays of fear and avoidance of the specifics of abuse or assault. This may be interpreted as disgust or other negative evaluation. Finally, we would emphasize that affective arousal is not in itself negative, and this needs to be recognized by therapist and client alike. In fact, the therapeutic situation may be the safest place in which to experience these feelings and have them validated.

To counter these potential barriers to disclosure, we preface our structured assessment questions with opening statements that accurately describe the circumstances in which sexual assault occurs, that establish the importance of our assessment task, and that indicate knowledge about the occurrence of sexual assault and its potential consequences. The following statement, taken from Saunders et al. (1989), provides an example.

One type of event that happens to men as well as women, and boys as well as girls, is sexual mistreatment or sexual assault. Men are assaulted under the same kinds of situations as women, but it may be even more difficult for a man to report an assault because he may be ashamed or fear that others will ridicule or not believe him. When asked about sexual abuse or mistreatment, many people tend to think about incidents in which they were attacked or mistreated by a total stranger. As you answer these questions, please remember that we need to know about all incidents of sexual abuse or mistreatment, not just those involving a stranger. Thus, please don't forget to tell us about incidents that might have happened when you were a child or those in which the person who tried to abuse or mistreat you was someone you knew, such as a friend, boyfriend or girlfriend, or even a spouse or family member. Now, here are some questions about some of these experiences you might have had. (p. 274)

DETERMINATION OF TYPE
OF SEXUAL ASSAULT

After establishing a supportive, nonjudgmental atmosphere, it is important to use behaviorally specific questions to obtain a history of all types of sexual assault incidents that have occurred (Kilpatrick, 1983). In our clinic, we routinely assess history of the following types of sexual assault incidents: (1) completed rape; (2) completed molestation; (3) attempted rape; and (4) attempted molestation. As noted earlier, findings indicate that completed rape is most likely to lead to PTSD, followed by completed molestation. Thus it is critical for the therapist to find out about the specific type of assault experienced.

A number of recently developed self-report and interview schedules are helpful in attempting to determine type of sexual assault (Koss & Gidycz, 1985; Kilpatrick, Best, et al., 1989). Included here as examples are the behaviorally specific items used by Kilpatrick, Best, et al. (1989) to determine whether a woman has ever experienced a completed rape:

Has a man or boy ever made you have sex by using force or threatening to harm you or someone close to you? Just so there is no mistake, by sex we mean putting a penis in your vagina.

Has anyone ever made you have oral sex by force or threat of harm? Just so there is no mistake, by oral sex we mean that a man or a boy put his penis in your mouth or someone penetrated your vagina or anus with their mouth or tongue.

Has anyone ever made you have anal sex by force or threat of harm?

Has anyone ever put fingers or objects in your vagina or anus against your will by using force or threats?

A positive response to any of the preceding items would indicate that a women has been a rape victim. Finally, Saunders et al. (1989) have developed a brief victimization screening questionnaire that includes items to assess whether a client has ever been the victim of a variety of sexual assault incidents. The items assessing sexual molestation are as follows:

> Have you ever had any experience in which someone tried to molest you sexually—that is, they made serious unwanted sexual advances but did not attempt full sexual relations?
>
> Have you ever been in a situation in which you were pressured into doing more sexually than you wanted to do; that is, a situation in which someone pressured you against your will into forced contact with the sexual parts of your body or their body? (p. 275)

TRAUMA-RELATED VARIABLES

Research findings support the significance of trauma-related variables in the development of sexual-assault-related PTSD. These include both objective characteristics of assault, such as receipt of injury, as well as cognitive appraisal variables, such as fear of being killed during assault (Kilpatrick, Saunders, et al., 1989).

Following procedures developed by Kilpatrick, Veronen, et al. (1987), in reference to each identified sexual assault we inquire about whether (1) the client was afraid of actual serious injury or death; and (2) whether and to what degree the client actually suffered injury. Other incident characteristics that we ask about include age at the time of victimization, relationship to the perpetrator, presence of a weapon, and chronicity (serial incidents vs. a single incident). On the basis of cognitive mediational models of PTSD, we also assess for presence of self-blame; changes in assumptions about the self, the world and others; and belief in personal invulnerability.

Other trauma-related variables that should be assessed for the purpose of clinical intervention include stimuli that have come to elicit a conditioned response subsequent to the initial trauma. These variables are discussed in detail in the "treatment" section of the chapter.

Assessment of Other Trauma History

A final historical variable that can influence the likelihood of PTSD development or maintenance in victims of sexual assault is the presence of a history of other traumatic events that in themselves can produce PTSD (Resnick, Kilpatrick, & Lipovsky, 1991). Results of epidemiological studies indicate that many people have experienced multiple sexual assaults (Burnam et al., 1988) and multiple types of traumatic events, including physical assault and other crimes, in addition to sexual assault (Kilpatrick, Saunders, et al., 1987; Kilpatrick, 1990). Clinically, those who have had long and complicated trauma histories, history of trauma occurring at potentially critical developmental stages, or prior onset of PTSD may display different symptom or adaptational profiles following sexual assault, and these profiles may require specialized treatment techniques. Moreover, in these cases treatment targeted at reducing PTSD symptoms associated with multiple traumas may be indicated. Thus, following assessment of the index sexual assault incident, we proceed to gather information about the client's entire history of traumatic events.

Assessment of the Symptom Domain

Symptom criteria for PTSD reflect a multiple-channel adaptation following trauma, with particular patterns of cognitive, behavioral, affective, and physiological modes of responding; these may be either responses to specific reminders of trauma or fairly chronic adaptations since trauma exposure. This assessment can best be accomplished by using multiple methods, including clinical interview, self-report instruments, behavioral observation, and physiological assessment. In addition, reports by family members or significant others of changes in behavior following trauma can be extremely useful. Before discussing these specific assessment techniques, we address the important issues of comorbidity and temporal course of PTSD.

COMORBIDITY

PTSD is not the only disorder that may occur following sexual assault. Sexual assault and rape have been associated with an increased risk of major depressive disorder, increased rates of suicidal ideation and attempts, other anxiety disorders, substance abuse (Frank & Anderson, 1987; Kilpatrick, Veronen, et al., 1987; Burnam et al., 1988), and sexual dysfunction (Becker, Skinner, Abel, & Treacy, 1982). In addition, high rates of comorbidity of PTSD with other psychiatric disorders have been observed in other community samples (Helzer, Robins, & McEvoy, 1987; Kilpatrick, Best, et al., 1989).

These data indicate that subjects with positive histories of sexual assault, and particularly those with assault-related PTSD, should be thoroughly evaluated for a variety of other psychological disorders as well. Assessment instruments that cover a broad array of symptomatology, including other anxiety symptoms, depression, and substance abuse, should be employed. The presence of comorbid conditions may dictate specific treatment approaches targeted at these disorders. In addition, the timing of behavioral treatment of PTSD symptoms may be affected (Keane, Fairbank, Caddell, & Zimering, 1989).

TEMPORAL FACTORS

Data on the natural course of PTSD indicate that the 3-month period after rape is a critical one. After 3 months, some victims recover while others display persistent distress (Rothbaum et al., 1990). The immediate postrape period may also relate to shifting patterns of symptoms. Kilpatrick et al. (1979) found that diffuse psychological distress decreased by the 3-month point, but that symptoms related to anxiety and specific assault-related fears persisted over time.

Close attention should be paid to clients' initial levels of distress and reports of their subjective distress at the time of assault, since data indicate that level of initial distress in the immediate aftermath of sexual assault (Rothbaum et al., 1990; Kilpatrick, Veronen, & Best, 1985) or at the time of the assault (Girelli, Resick, Marhoefer-Dvorak, & Hutter, 1986) is a significant predictor of chronic distress following sexual assault. These findings also indicate that assessment should be conducted at repeated intervals. Moreover, the data have implications for evaluations of treatment efficacy: On the basis of the finding that the 3 months after rape may be a critical time period in which a large number of victims show improvement in PTSD and general distress, evaluations of treatment efficacy should be conducted with clients who are at least 3 months past the rape (Kilpatrick & Calhoun, 1988).

Finally, length of time since trauma or time since onset of chronic PTSD may be associated with different patterns of adaptation that need to be addressed in both assessment and treatment. It has been suggested that those with chronic PTSD may have more diffuse problems in some areas such as social adjustment, and that these may require specialized treatment approaches (Keane et al., 1989). It is possible that impairment in social, vocational and other areas of adjustment may reflect adaptation to the presence of PTSD as well as to a history of trauma.

Specific Assessment Methods and Measures

STRUCTURED DIAGNOSTIC INTERVIEWS

Several structured diagnostic interviews are available for the assessment of PTSD; they provide probe questions to be used to elicit responses from the subject in reference to all PTSD symptoms. Major interview schedules include the Structured Clinical Interview for DSM-III-R (SCID; Spitzer, Williams, & Gibbon, 1987); the Diagnostic Interview Schedule (Robins, Helzer, Croughan, & Ratcliff, 1981); the Anxiety Disorders Interview Schedule (Blanchard, Gerardi, Kolb, & Barlow, 1986); and the Clinician Administered PTSD Scale—Form 1 (Blake et al., 1990).

In our clinic, we have modified the SCID by incorporating the thorough trauma assessment described above. Once a thorough screening for traumatic events has been completed, we conduct the SCID to assess PTSD symptoms in reference to the specific events the client has experienced. In asking about each symptom, we assess whether it occurred after each victimization or trauma and, when applicable, whether the content of the symptom (e.g., nightmares) related to specific trauma(s) experienced. This procedure allows us to gather information about the developmental history of PTSD, and to evaluate the need for treatment of distress associated with specific traumas in a client's history (Resnick et al., 1991). In addition to our initial evaluation using the SCID, we administer a weekly checklist during treatment to assess progress in reduction of PTSD symptoms (see Figure 5.1). The items are adapted from the SCID phrasing. Subjects are asked how many days each particular symptom occurred in the past week. This yields summary scores for reexperiencing, avoidance, and increased arousal, as well as for total PTSD symptoms.

PSYCHOMETRIC ASSESSMENT INSTRUMENTS

At the end of the first assessment session, clients complete a standard battery of self-report instruments. These instruments tap intensity of current PTSD symptoms and are also used to indicate areas of general psychological distress (e.g., depression) that may require more in-depth assessment. The measures described here are routinely administered before and after treatment to evaluate client progress. Non-trauma-specific measures include the Symptom Checklist 90—Revised (SCL-90-R; Derogatis, 1977) and the Beck Depression Inventory (Beck, Ward, Mendelson, Mock, & Erbaugh, 1961). In addition to the general utility

For each item mark number of days that each symptom occurred in past week.

B1.   Frequent distressing thoughts or memories of event (sometimes even without reminders)
B2.   Distressing dreams of the event
B3.   Sudden acting or feeling as if the event were happening again, or flashbacks (Circle): seeing   hearing   smelling   physically feeling parts of what happened
B4.   Reminders of what happened (cues, anniversaries, physical locations, etc.) Record last reminder

C1.   Deliberate efforts to avoid thoughts or feelings about the event
C2.   Deliberate efforts to avoid activities or situations that remind you of the event
C3.   Difficulty remembering some part of the event
C4.   Decreased interest in activities you used to enjoy
C5.   Feeling cut off from others
C6   Feeling numb or unable to have loving feelings for others
C7.   Feeling that you might die young, or that other bad things will happen to you

D1.   Difficulty falling or staying asleep
D2.   Irritability or outbursts of anger
D3.   Difficulty concentrating
D4.   Being watchful or on guard
D5.   Jumpiness or being easily startled
D6.   Physical reactions to reminders of event
      Circle: heart beats faster   sweating   shaking   changes in breathing
      Example of last physical reaction:

FIGURE 5.1.   Weekly symptom checklist.

of the SCL-90-R, a Crime-Related PTSD subscale of the SCL-90-R has been developed that yields a cutoff score for PTSD; we currently use this subscale in our clinic (Saunders, Mandoki, & Kilpatrick, 1990).

Other trauma-specific measures that we use include the Impact of Event Scale (IES; Horowitz, Wilner, & Alvarez, 1979) and the Rape Aftermath Symptom Test (RAST; Kilpatrick, 1988). The IES is useful as a measure of intensity of current intrusive and avoidance symptoms of PTSD, whereas the RAST assesses the degree of current fear associated with trauma-related stimuli, as well as more general anxiety-related symptoms. Preliminary data support the clinical utility of the IES and RAST for either prediction (Rothbaum et al., 1990) or detection of PTSD (Resnick et al., 1991).

PSYCHOPHYSIOLOGICAL ASSESSMENT

Although we do not conduct psychophysiological assessment as part of our standard evaluation, we briefly review the potential use of these procedures. Indices of psychophysiological arousal have been found to be very specific indicators of PTSD in studies of combat veterans assessed either at baseline or in response to trauma-related cues (Malloy, Fairbank, & Keane, 1983; Blanchard, Kolb, Pallmeyer, & Gerardi, 1982; Pitman, Orr, Forgue, de Jong, & Claiborn, 1987). Thus, positive indication of arousal can add to the convergent validity of diagnosis. In addition, these indices provide more objective data than interview or self-report measures, and can be used to monitor progress in treatment.

Very few published data exist about psychophysiological responses of sexual assault victims under neutral or stressor conditions, aside from several treatment case studies (Rychtarik, Silverman, Van Landingham, & Prue, 1984; Kilpatrick & Amick, 1985; Blanchard & Abel, 1976). Interestingly, in all cases there were reductions in at least some measures of arousal from initial elevations observed, despite the variety of treatment methods employed. The treatment methods used in the three studies were implosion, stress inoculation training, and biofeedback, respectively. These findings indicate that at least in cases where there is initial evidence of arousal, psychophysiological measures may be useful in monitoring treatment outcome.

Treatment

Major goals of therapy for sexual-assault-related PTSD are (1) reducing anxiety related to conditioned stimuli that are objectively nonthreatening; and (2) altering perceived threat related to physiological, affective, and cognitive responses associated with the traumatic memory. In addition, cognitive therapy is useful to facilitate adaptive appraisal of the causality of sexual assault, including issues of responsibility and blame. These issues are important for helping clients revise their assumptions about the safety and controllability of events, self-worth, and future expectations.

The two cognitive–behavioral approaches most frequently applied to PTSD are exposure techniques and coping skills treatments (Fairbank & Brown, 1987). In a review of the use of exposure therapy in treatment of anxiety disorder, Foa and Kozak (1986) have suggested that this technique allows for access to and modification of fear structures associated with trauma; as they see it, the threat interpretations and negative valence associated with stimuli and responses are modified through the reduction in anxiety within and across repeated exposure trials. Steketee and Foa (1987) have suggested that coping skills techniques such as relaxation training may promote dissociation between physiological arousal and stimuli that previously elicited fear. Finally, cognitive restructuring techniques, which may be considered within the rubric of coping skills training, may directly alter appraisal of events through provision of corrective information and education.

Stress Inoculation Training

The treatment program used at the Crime Victims Research and Treatment Center includes a combination of primarily skills training and exposure-based techniques. This program, called stress inoculation training (SIT), was developed by Veronen and Kilpatrick (1983) to treat primary symptoms presented by rape victims. The SIT regimen contains an initial educational phase, followed by training in sets of coping skills that specifically address anxiety-related symptoms in the physiological, cognitive, and behavioral channels. Over the course of approximately 12 to 14 sessions of weekly treatment, clients are instructed to apply each set of skills, individually and in combination, to confront previously avoided fear-eliciting situations. Because of the importance of anxiety reduction within sessions, 90 minute sessions may be optimal unless a client is able to achieve relative relaxation earlier. Progression through the different skills application phases can be modified according to clients' progress and particular needs. Typically, at least two sessions are required for mastery of each skill.

EDUCATIONAL PHASE

In the first two sessions, each client is presented with a learning-based explanation of fears related to rape trauma, as well as an explanation of the ways anxiety is expressed in the physiological, cognitive, and behavioral channels (Lang, 1968). This is followed by provision of a rationale for treatment using SIT. The learning theory model is presented in lay language, and the client is also given a handout to read that presents the model and describes typical reactions to sexual assault. Sexual assault is described as an emergency of situation that is often (or at least is perceived as) life-threatening or extremely dangerous. It is suggested that, in this type of situation, responses are automatic, without any prior learning required. The types of automatic reactions are then described as occurring in three response channels: (1) physical reactions; (2)

thoughts focused on threat; and (3) survival behaviors that may include freezing, fighting, or attempting to flee. The client is then asked to describe his or her own reactions during the sexual assault.

It is explained that in this type of "automatic" situation, objects, people, and types of activities that were paired with the assault can come to bring about reactions in the three response channels because they have become learned signals of danger. In other words, the client did not respond in these ways to these cues prior to assault. The therapist then asks the client to give examples of stimuli that have come to elicit fear. Three target fears are identified, and these become goals for treatment. These stimuli often include time of day, physical locations, people with physical characteristics similar to those of the assailant, and sexual and interpersonal activities. The client is asked to relate current responses to these cues in the three major channels, and parallels are drawn with the original traumatic situation and responses.

Principles of stimulus generalization and higher-order conditioning are also explained. As an example of higher-order conditioning, the therapist explains that the therapy situation can become a cue for anxiety because it is paired with talking and thinking about the assault. The client is told that this is expected on the basis of the learning theory model. The client is then asked about levels of discomfort in the therapy session, and future anxiety is predicted. However, it is also predicted that anxiety will decrease over time and in future sessions as part of the natural course of repeated experiences in which trauma does not recur.

Finally, the role of avoidance in maintaining sexual-assault-related anxiety is explicated. The client is taught that avoidance of learned cues does reduce anxiety in the short run, and thus it works for that purpose. The drawbacks are also reviewed, including prevention of mastery experiences, perpetuation of fear, and undesirable restrictions in lifestyle. SIT is then presented as a treatment program to teach more effective coping strategies so that clients are able to overcome their fears and successfully function in previously distressing situations. A preview is given of the types of skills taught, including relaxation techniques, and cognitive and behavioral coping strategies.

The client is taught that responses in one channel may set off responses in other channels. For example, a physical reaction may lead to assault-related thoughts, and the reverse relationship may also apply. It is suggested that if responses are identified early enough and managed, a "full-blown" anxiety response may be prevented. However, the client is also instructed that the goal of treatment is not the elimination of anxiety. Anxiety is described as functional and as having a natural time course. Thus, if an anxiety reaction occurs in an objectively nonthreatening situation, the client is told that the affect is not to be avoided. Instructions are given (1) to expect that it may escalate but that it will also naturally decrease; and (2) to remain in the situation long enough for the anxiety to decrease, in order to regain control over the feared situation.

A second element in SIT education includes presenting accurate information about sexual assault crimes and issues of responsibility and safety. This is important so that a client can reassess self-blame attributions about the assault and develop a greater sense of control in the environment. For example, many clients are unaware of the prevalence of sexual assault and the circumstances in which it occurs. These circumstances directly counter many myths about sexual assault that lead to self-blame. Because of myths about rape, such as the notion that a woman deserves to be assaulted if she dresses in a certain way, or that sexual assault is perpetrated only by strangers, it is very important to assess each client's views about responsibility and to provide this corrective information.

We emphasize to all clients that whatever they did to survive assault was good and cannot be second-guessed. In addition, we acknowledge that being assaulted by a known individual is more common than stranger rape and can be an extremely frightening situation that violates previous assumptions of safety and trust. Finally, we emphasize that the bottom line of responsibility is that a perpetrator has no right to commit an assault, no matter what the circumstances are. In cases of child sexual assault, it is emphasized that even if children have offered assent, they are not considered as having the capability to make that type of decision and that it is up to adults to protect the children from harm, including sexual abuse or assault. Another helpful tactic to address issues of self–blame is to clarify with the client the distinction between intent prior to assault and outcome. This elicits the realization that the client did not intend to be assaulted or to put himself or herself in a vulnerable position.

For personal safety issues, it is acknowledged that sexual assault is a frequently occurring event, but that actions can be taken to promote safety. These include reporting to police, having a safety check conducted on doors, locks, and windows, and paying attention to cues in the environment that signal relatively lower risk of assault. These cues can include being out in public among groups of people and staying in well-lit areas. Following assault, a client may overlook these signals in the environment and may need to reappraise and learn safety cues.

We recommend that family members or significant others be included in the educational phase of treatment, so that they have a basis for understanding the persistence of anxiety even though the assault situation is over. In addition, when family members understand the treatment rationale, they can help the client complete homework assignments.

SKILLS ACQUISITION AND APPLICATION

As in behavioral treatment for other anxiety disorders, separate skills are applied for the three channels in which anxiety may be expressed. Two techniques are taught in each channel to offer clients some choice, based on what is most effective or preferred. All skills are practiced with the therapist in session and between sessions. Each technique is first applied to a non-assault-related stressor, followed by use of the technique with a sexual-assault-related stressor. At the beginning of each session, progress with homework assignments is reviewed.

Controlled Breathing. We start anxiety management training in the physiological channel with instruction in deep breathing. Clients are taught to calm themselves down by taking even breaths and slowly exhaling over repeated trials. In session, a client and therapist practice controlled diaphragmatic breathing at a rate of approximately 3 to 4 seconds each for inhaling and exhaling. This is repeated for at least 20 breaths. In subsequent sessions, clients are also directed to use imagery of a self-selected scene in which they feel safe and comfortable as they control their breathing. For homework, clients are instructed to practice the controlled breathing skill daily. They are first instructed to practice this skill in either a non-stress-related situation or a non-assault-related stressful situation, such as test anxiety. Following this application, they are instructed to apply the skill with an assault-related situation, such as being home alone.

Deep Muscle Relaxation. The second technique in the physiological channel is Jacobsonian muscle relaxation (Jacobson, 1938). At least one entire session is set aside for the sole purpose of achieving muscle relaxation in the therapy setting. The instructions for tensing and relaxing all major muscle groups are tape-recorded for home practice. Clients are instructed that muscle relaxation can promote a reduction in general level of anxiety if it is practiced regularly. Homework includes practicing the procedure at least once daily.

Cognitive Restructuring. After practicing controlled breathing, a client is asked to relate to the therapist the details of the sexual assault, to the degree that the client is comfortable doing so. It is important to allow a sufficient amount of time in this session for the client to experience a decrease in anxiety prior to leaving the therapist's office. We typically set aside at least 90 minutes. During the account of the event, the therapist probes to elicit reactions across channels in response to elements of the assault. Issues of self-blame are again addressed, and learning principles that illustrate connections between current fears and reactions with assault experiences are again discussed. This retelling of the event is often essential for identifying specific target fears and for providing constructive feedback about assigned responsibility for the assault. In addition, retelling the trauma may also provide a decrease in anxiety associated with the memory of the sexual assault. Over the course of relating the incident, clients are asked to report "subjective units of discomfort" (SUDs) ratings.

At the end of the retelling portion of the session, controlled breathing is again practiced. The number of sessions needed to conduct this focused processing of the memory of the sexual assault varies. The general criteria are that the client should be able to discuss the event in detail without significant avoidance of memory content, and should demonstrate a reduction in all important cognitive distortions related to predictability, controllability, and threat. This component of treatment potentially involves some imaginal exposure, but it is not generally conducted repeatedly, as with flooding, over the course of several sessions. The major goals are obtaining information about specific cues and actively providing corrective information. However, it could be argued that once the incident has been related in detail even on one occasion, exposure to the memory continues in other sessions about the assault— albeit less directly, in the context of the skills training components of SIT.

Thought Stopping.   In the cognitive channel, the techniques of thought stopping (Wolpe, 1958) and guided self-dialogue (Meichenbaum, 1974) are taught. Thought stopping is demonstrated by having the client form a non-assault-related thought, then signal nonverbally to the therapist when the thought is clearly in mind. At this time the therapist says "Stop!" loudly and claps. This technique is practiced with the client verbalizing "Stop!" first aloud and then silently. In the use of thought stopping, a distinction is made between productive processing of the event, which is framed as a natural part of recovery, and ruminative self-statements that are distressing. Examples of nonproductive self-statements are repetitive thoughts such as "I am a bad person" or "I am going to faint in public." The client is instructed that thought stopping is designed to provide immediate control of these nonproductive thoughts.

To address the negative thoughts in therapy, the therapist must first elicit from the client specific cognitions that can be objectively evaluated. For example, probes to the statement "I am a bad person" might relate to events surrounding the assault. The validity of negative interpretations can then be evaluated. Similarly, probes to the fainting statement might focus on both specific factors that lead to the expectation of fainting, as well as fears related to anticipated consequences of fainting. Again, once the important cognitions are made explicit in the therapy session, their validity can be examined.

Guided Self-Dialogue. Guided self-dialogue (Meichenbaum, 1974) includes assessing irrational or dysfunctional cognitions and replacing them with more functional cognitions that promote confronting and coping with a stressor. Several adaptive self-statements are taught for each phase of coping with a stressor event. Phases of coping are defined as preparation, confrontation, management of affect, and reinforcement after taking action. For example, preparation includes problem identification, as well as realistic appraisal of negative outcome. Confrontation includes breaking down the goal into manageable steps, concentrating on what needs to be done at each step, and use of encouraging statements. Statements for managing affect include a focus on anxiety as manageable and time-limited.

It is suggested that early signals of anxiety be used as a sign to employ coping skills. In addition, the possibility of becoming overwhelmed or experiencing an extreme escalation of arousal is raised. It is suggested that in this situation, decatastrophizing statements be used that emphasize the absence of objective threat and the natural time course of anxiety and arousal. Finally, it is important for clients to be able to integrate positive information about coping with a stressor and to reinforce themselves for doing so. Veronen and Kilpatrick (1983) suggest the use of index cards on which a client can record self-statements for each phase of coping. Again, both of these techniques are applied in relation to non-assault-related and assault-related stressors.

Role Playing. The techniques of role playing and covert modeling are applied to address behavioral avoidance aspects. Role playing is practiced in session until the client can successfully demonstrate the desired behavior. Typically, the therapist first models the desired behavior and then the roles are switched. As Veronen and Kilpatrick note in their guidelines, (1983) it is important to give clients feedback on their nonverbal as well as verbal performance. Important nonverbal performance elements include posture, tone of voice, and facial expression. Often role plays involve interpersonal situations, and many clients require education about techniques of assertion as well. For example, a client may choose the assault-related problem of being uncomfortable about a specific sexual behavior with his or her sexual partner. Assertive communication about sexual issues may be new to the client. Thus, education about the importance of identifying and communicating feelings and the right to communicate them is essential. Homework entails actually carrying out the practiced interaction.

Covert Modeling. Covert modeling involves imaginal successful progression through an anxiety-producing situation. As suggested by Veronen and Kilpatrick (1983), this technique can be explained to clients as being like role playing conducted in imagination. An example of this is having a client imagine attending a meeting with the district attorney. In imagery, rehearsal can include each step the client would take: preparing for the meeting: anticipating an increase in affective arousal; successfully using coping skills to manage arousal or self-statements to deal with feelings of being overwhelmed; completing the task; and providing self-reinforcement following the task, through either self-statements or rewarding activities.

TREATMENT EFFICACY

Several single-case reports support the efficacy of SIT in reducing symptoms of fear, anxiety, negative mood state, and PTSD symptoms (Veronen & Kilpatrick, 1983; Kilpatrick & Amick, 1985). The results of the first group comparison study (Resick, Jordan, Girelli, Hutter, & Marhoefer-Dvorak, 1988) indicated that a group receiving SIT showed significant improvement in anxiety-related symptoms when compared to a no-treatment control group. However, the results for SIT were not significantly different from those for either assertion training or supportive–educational therapy conditions.

Rothbaum and Foa (in press) have conducted a study to assess the relative efficacy of skills training (SIT) versus prolonged exposure techniques for treatment of PTSD with rape victims. However, in contrast to the guidelines of Veronen and Kilpatrick (1983), any imaginal or *in vivo* exposure elements were omitted from the SIT condition, in order to clarify differential effects of the two major behavioral treatments. The prolonged exposure condition included imaginal exposure to the memory of the rape assault, as well as *in vivo* exposure homework. Preliminary results (Dancu & Foa, in press) indicated that both SIT and exposure were superior to supportive counseling and control groups immediately after treatment, with the SIT group displaying greatest improvement. However, at 3-month follow-up, there was a greater problem with relapse in the SIT condition than in to the exposure condition.

These findings illustrate the preliminary nature of current knowledge about relative efficacy of behavioral treatments for PTSD. Accordingly, Foa and her colleagues are currently conducting a study comparing a combined SIT and exposure treatment approach to separate SIT and exposure conditions. This study should yield useful information about the combined use of skills and exposure-based approaches.

Future Directions for Integrating Behavioral Approaches

It may be the case that prolonged exposure and SIT are relatively more effective in treating different components of PTSD. If this is the case, an integrated approach combining elements of the two treatments may be optimal. One possible limitation of SIT as currently conducted is that clients are not necessarily inoculated to deal with extremely high levels of arousal. For example, clients may be successful at managing anxiety on many occasions by using a variety of skills, but in instances where management is unsuccessful a client may not be well prepared to deal with it and may panic.

In contrast, prolonged exposure allows clients to learn that extreme levels of arousal are not dangerous and that arousal will decrease over time. However, exposure techniques such as flooding lead to initial increases in symptomatology, which sometimes require a more controlled treatment environment. In addition, some therapists may be afraid of dealing with the intense levels of arousal in initial sessions of prolonged exposure to traumatic memories. Finally, particularly for clients whose symptom patterns are chronic, avoidance may have led to skills deficits that are not ameliorated by prolonged exposure treatment. In some of these cases, a coping skills approach may provide necessary tools for mastery of situations previously avoided. Thus, the two treatment approaches might be usefully combined in the treatment of PTSD.

One such program that integrates anxiety management and exposure to somatic cues has been used successfully in the treatment of other anxiety disorders by Barlow and his colleagues (Barlow & Craske, 1990). This comprehensive approach might be a very useful model for treatment of PTSD as well. The approach emphasizes skills acquisition in the early treatment sessions, to reduce general anxiety and increase the threshold at which panic occurs. Once the exposure phase of treatment is reached, clients are encouraged to elicit as much arousal as possible and to employ anxiety management techniques only when the exercises are complete. Thus, the program provides a framework for complementary use of the two approaches.

The exposure component included in Barlow and Craske's (1990) treatment program differs in an important way from that usually used in treating PTSD. It emphasizes exposure to somatic cues that signal panic and that are components of panic attacks (hyperventilation, dizziness, muscle tension, etc.). Exposure in session is accomplished by eliciting somatic cues; for instance, hyperventilation is induced by having the client deliberately breathe deeply and rapidly. In the natural environment, such situations as physical activity are used to produce somatic sensations. Along with this exposure, clients learn that these reactions are actually nonthreatening.

In contrast, present exposure treatments for PTSD have primarily involved presentation of cognitive stimulus cues such as images and memories, which then elicit arousal. Since response elements of traumatic memories are thought to be important links to current fear and avoidance responses, exposure to somatic cues might also be helpful in treating PTSD. In fact, the use of exposure to somatic cues prior to exposure to traumatic memories might be seen as consistent with both SIT and prolonged exposure treatments. As with SIT, rather than exposing the client to cognitive and physiological cues at once, exposure could be conducted first with somatic sensations; this would give the client a sense of mastery, and would allow both therapist and client to be less afraid of physiological reactions when the client is processing traumatic memories. Once exposure to somatic cues has been conducted, exposure to the combination of cognitive and physiological cues could be conducted to allow for successful processing of traumatic memories.

References

Atkeson, B. M., Calhoun, K. S., Resick, P. A., & Ellis, E. M. (1982). Victims of rape: Repeated assessment of depressive symptoms. *Journal of Consulting and Clinical Psychology, 50*, 96–102.

Barlow, D. H., & Craske, M. G. (1990). *Mastery of your anxiety and panic (MAP)*. Albany: Center for Stress and Anxiety Disorders, State University of New York at Albany, Graywind Press.

Beck, A. T., Ward, C. H., Mendelson, M., Mock, J., & Erbaugh, J. (1961). An inventory for measuring depression. *Archives of General Psychiatry, 4*, 561–571.

Beck, J. C., & van der Kolk, B. (1987). Reports of childhood incest and current behavior of chronically hospitalized psychotic women. *American Journal of Psychiatry, 144*, 1474–1476.

Becker, J. V., Skinner, L. J., Abel, G. G., & Treacy, E. C. (1982). Incidence and types of sexual dysfunctions in rape and incest victims. *Journal of Sex and Marital Therapy, 8*, 65–74.

Blake, D. D., Weathers, F. W., Nagy, L. M., Kaloupek, D. G., Klauminzer, G., Charney, & Keane, T. M. (1990). A clinician rating scale for assessing current and lifetime PTSD: The CAPS–1. *the Behavior Therapist, 13*, 187–188.

Blanchard, E. B., & Abel, G. (1976). An experimental case study of the biofeedback treatment of a rape-induced psychophysiological cardiovascular disorder. *Behavior Therapy, 7*, 113–119.

Blanchard, E. B., Gerardi, R. J., Kolb, L. C., & Barlow, D. H. (1986). The utility of the Anxiety Disorders Interview Schedule (ADIS) in the diagnosis of post-traumatic stress disorder (PTSD) in Vietnam veterans. *Behaviour Research and Therapy, 24*, 577–580.

Blanchard, E. B., Kolb, L. C., Pallmeyer, T. P., & Gerardi, R. J. (1982). The development of a psychophysiological assessment procedure for PTSD in Vietnam veterans. *Psychiatric Quarterly, 54*, 220–228.

Bryer, J. B., Nelson, B. A., Miller, J. B., & Krol, P. A. (1987). Childhood sexual and physical abuse as factors in adult psychiatric illness. *American Journal of Psychiatry, 144*, 1426–1430.

Burnam, M. A., Stein, J. A., Golding, J. M., Siegel, J. M., Sorenson, S. B., Forsythe, A. B., & Telles, C. A. (1988). Sexual assault and mental disorders in a community population. *Journal of Consulting and Clinical Psychology, 56*, 843–850.

Dancu, C. V., & Foa, E. B. (in press). Cognitive behavior therapy with post-traumatic stress disorder. In A. Freeman & F. M. Dattilio (Eds.), *Casebook in cognitive behavior therapy*. New York: Plenum.

Derogatis, L. R. (1977). *SCL-90: Administration, scoring and procedure manual-I for the R (revised) version*. Baltimore: Johns Hopkins University School of Medicine.

Fairbank, J. A., & Brown, T. A. (1987). Current behavioral approaches to the treatment of posttraumatic stress disorder. *the Behavior Therapist, 3*, 57–64.

Foa, E. B., & Kozak, M. J. (1986). Emotional processing of fear: Exposure to corrective information. *Psychological Bulletin, 99*, 20–35.

Foa, E. B., Steketee, G., & Rothbaum, B. O. (1989). Behavioral/cognitive conceptualizations of post-traumatic stress disorder. *Behavior Therapy, 20*, 155–176.

Foy, D. W., Osato, S. S., Houskamp, B. M., & Neumann, D. A. (in press). PTSD etiology. In P. A. Saigh (Ed.), *Posttraumatic stress disorder: Behavioral assessment and treatment*. Elmsford, NY: Maxwell Press.

Frank, E., & Anderson, B. P. (1987). Psychiatric disorders in rape victims: Past history and current symptomatology. *Comprehensive Psychiatry, 28*, 77–82.

Frank, E., Turner, S. M., & Duffy, B. (1979). Depressive symptoms in rape victims. *Journal of Affective Disorders, 1*, 269–277.

Girelli, S. A., Resick, P. A., Marhoefer-Dvorak, S., & Hutter, C. K. (1986). Subjective distress and violence during rape: Their effects on long-term fear. *Victims and Violence, 1*, 35–46.

Helzer, J. E., Robins, L. N., & McEvoy, L. (1987). Post-traumatic stress disorder in the general population. *New England Journal of Medicine, 317*, 1630–1634.

Horowitz, M., Wilner, N., & Alvarez, W. (1979). Impact of Event Scale: A measure of subjective stress. *Psychosomatic Medicine, 41*(3), 209–218.

Jacobson, A., & Richardson, B. (1987). Assault experiences of 100 psychiatric inpatients: Evidence of the need for routine inquiry. *American Journal of Psychiatry*, *144*, 908–913.

Jacobson, E. (1938). *Progressive relaxation*. Chicago: University of Chicago Press.

Janoff-Bulman, R. (1985). The aftermath of victimization: Rebuilding shattered assumptions. In C. R. Figley (Ed.), *Trauma and its wake: Vol. 1. The study and treatment of posttraumatic stress disorders* (pp. 15–35). New York: Brunner/ Mazel.

Jones, J. C., & Barlow, D. H. (1990). The etiology of posttraumatic stress disorder. *Clinical Psychology Review*, *10*, 299–328.

Keane, T. M., Fairbank, J. A., Caddell, J. M., & Zimering, R. T. (1989). Implosive (flooding) therapy reduces symptoms of PTSD in Vietnam combat veterans. *Behavior Therapy*, *20*, 245–260.

Keane, T. M., Wolfe, J., & Taylor, K. L. (1987). Posttraumatic stress disorder: Evidence for diagnostic validity and methods of psychological assessment. *Journal of Clinical Psychology*, *43*, 32–43.

Kilpatrick, D. G. (1983). Rape victims: Detection, assessment, and treatment. *The Clinical Psychologist*, *36*(4), 92–95.

Kilpatrick, D. G. (1988). Rape Aftermath Symptom Test. In M. Hersen & A. S. Bellack (Eds.), *Dictionary of behavioral assessment techniques* (pp. 366–367). Elmsford, NY: Pergamon Press.

Kilpatrick, D. G. (1990, October). The epidemiology of potentially stressful events and their traumatic impact: Implications for prevention. In C. Dunning (Chair), *Trauma studies: Contributions to prevention*. Plenary session conducted at the 6th Annual Meeting of the International Society for Traumatic Stress Studies, New Orleans.

Kilpatrick, D. G., & Amick, A. E. (1985). Rape trauma. In M. Hersen & C. G. Last (Eds.), *Behavior therapy casebook* (pp. 86–103). New York: Springer.

Kilpatrick, D. G., & Best, C. L. (1990, April). *Sexual assault victims: Data from a random national probability sample*. Paper presented at the 36th Annual Meeting of the Southeastern Psychological Association, Atlanta.

Kilpatrick, D. G., Best, C., Amick-McMullan, A., Saunders, B. E., Sturgis, E., Resnick, H. S., & Veronen, L. J. (1989, November). Criminal victimization, post-traumatic stress disorder, and substance abuse: A prospective study. In F. R. Abueg (Chair), *Co-morbidity in traumatic stress disorders with special attention to substance abuse and dependence*. Symposium conducted at the 23rd Annual Convention of the Association for Advancement of Behavior Therapy, Washington, DC.

Kilpatrick, D. G., & Calhoun, K. S. (1988). Early behavioral treatment for rape trauma: Efficacy or artifact? *Behavior Therapy*, *19*, 421–427.

Kilpatrick, D. G., Saunders, B. E., Amick-McMullan, A., Best, C. L., Veronen, L. J., & Resnick, H. S. (1989). Victim and crime factors associated with the development of crime-related post-traumatic stress disorder. *Behavior Therapy*, *20*, 199–214.

Kilpatrick, D.G., Saunders, B.E., Veronen, L.J., Best, C.L., & Von, J.M. (1987). Criminal victimization: Lifetime prevalence, reporting to police, and psychological impact. *Crime and Delinquency*, *33*(4), 479–489.

Kilpatrick, D. G., Veronen, L. J., & Best, C. L. (1985). Factors predicting psychological distress among rape victims. In C. R. Figley (Ed.), *Trauma and its wake: Vol. 1.*

The study and treatment of posttraumatic stress disorder (pp. 113–141). New York: Brunner/Mazel.

Kilpatrick, D. G., Veronen, L. J., & Resick, P. A. (1979). Assessment of the aftermath of rape: Changing patterns of fear. *Journal of Behavioral Assessment, 1*, 133–148.

Kilpatrick, D. G., Veronen, L. J., Saunders, B. E., Best, C. L., Amick-McMullan, A., & Paduhovich, J. (1987). *The psychological impact of crime: A study of randomly surveyed crime victims* (Final Report, Grant No. 84-IJ-CX-0039). Washington, DC: National Institute of Justice.

Koss, M. P., & Gidycz, C. A. (1985). Sexual Experiences Survey: Reliability and validity. *Journal of Consulting and Clinical Psychology, 53*, 422–423.

Koss, M. P., Gidycz, C. A., & Wisniewski, N. (1987). The scope of rape: Incidence and prevalence of sexual aggression and victimization in a national sample of higher education students. *Journal of Consulting and Clinical Psychology, 55*, 162–170.

Lang, P. J. (1968). Fear reduction and fear behavior: Problems in treating a construct. *Research in Psychotherapy, 3*, 90–102.

Malloy, P. F., Fairbank, J. A., & Keane, T. M. (1983). Validation of a multimethod assessment of posttraumatic stress disorders in Vietnam veterans. *Journal of Consulting and Clinical Psychology, 51*, 488–494.

Meichenbaum, D. (1974). *Cognitive behavior modification*. Morristown, NJ: General Learning Press.

Pitman, R. K., Orr, S. P., Forgue, D. F., de Jong, J. B., & Claiborn, J. M. (1987). Psychophysiologic assessment of posttraumatic stress disorder imagery in Vietnam combat veterans. *Archives of General Psychiatry, 44*, 970–975.

Resick, P. A., Jordan, C. G., Girelli, S. A., Hutter, C. K., & Marhoefer-Dvorak, S. (1988). A comparative outcome study of behavioral group therapy for sexual assault victims. *Behavior Therapy, 19*, 385–401.

Resnick, H. S., Kilpatrick, D. G., & Lipovsky, J. A. (1991). Assessment of rape-related posttraumatic stress disorder: Stressor and symptom dimensions. *Psychological Assessment, 3*, 561–572.

Robins, L. N., Helzer, J. E., Croughan, J., & Ratcliff, K. S. (1981) National Institute of Mental Health Diagnostic Interview Schedule: Its history, characteristics, and validity. *Archives of General Psychiatry, 38*, 381–389.

Rothbaum, B. O., & Foa, E. B. (in press). Cognitive–behavioral treatment of posttraumatic stress disorder. In P. A. Saigh (Ed.), *Posttraumatic stress disorder: Behavioral assessment and treatment*. Elmsford, NY: Maxwell Press.

Rothbaum, B. O., Foa, E. B., Riggs, D. S., Murdock, T., & Walsh, W. (in press). A prospective examination of post-traumatic stress disorder in rape victims. *Journal of Traumatic Stress.*

Rychtarik, R. G., Silverman, W. K., Van Landingham, W. P., & Prue, D. M. (1984). Treatment of an incest victim with implosive therapy: A case study. *Behavior Therapy, 15*, 410–420.

Saunders, B. E, Kilpatrick, D. G., Resnick, H. S., & Tidwell, R. P. (1989). Brief screening for lifetime history of criminal victimization at mental health intake: A preliminary study. *Journal of Interpersonal Violence, 4*(3), 267–277.

Saunders, B. E., Mandoki, K. A., & Kilpatrick, D. G. (1990). Development of a crime-related post-traumatic stress disorder scale within the Symptom Checklist-90—Revised. *Journal of Traumatic Stress, 3*, 439–448.

Spitzer, R. L., Williams, J. B. W., & Gibbon, M. (1987). *Structured Clinical Interview for DSM-III-R: Non-patient version* (SCID-NP-V). New York: New York State Psychiatric Institute.

Steketee, G., & Foa, E. B. (1987). Rape victims: Post-traumatic stress responses and their treatment. *Journal of Anxiety Disorders, 1,* 69–86.

Veronen, L. J., & Kilpatrick, D. G. (1983). Stress management for rape victims. In D. Meichenbaum & M. E. Jaremko (Eds.), *Stress reduction and prevention* (pp. 341–374). New York: Plenum.

Wolpe, J. (1958). *Psychotherapy by reciprocal inhibition.* Stanford, CA: Stanford University Press.

6

Assessment and Treatment of Post-Traumatic Stress Disorder in Child Survivors of Sexual Assault

JULIE A. LIPOVSKY

Most research on PTSD to date has addressed the etiology, prevalence, and treatment of the disorder in adults. However, early reports of children's responses to traumatic events bear close resemblance to current diagnostic symptoms of PTSD (e.g., Bloch, Silber, & Perry, 1956; Titchener & Kapp, 1976). More recent studies of children's psychological reactions (Burke, Borus, Burns, Millstein, & Beasley, 1982; Dollinger, O'Donnell, & Staley, 1984) also suggest that children exposed to traumatic events develop symptom patterns indicative of PTSD.

Most recently, studies of PTSD in children have examined children exposed to natural disaster (Frederick, 1985; Earls, Smith, Reich, & Jung, 1988), man-made disaster (Handford et al., 1986), war-related trauma (Arroyo & Eth, 1985; Kinzie, Sack, Angell, Manson, & Rath, 1986; Saigh, 1987a), violent crime (e.g., Malmquist, 1986; Pynoos et al., 1987; Pynoos & Nader, 1988; Nader, Pynoos, Fairbanks, & Frederick, 1990), a ferry disaster (Yule & Williams, 1990), and trauma related to medical procedures (Stoddard, Norman, Murphy, & Beardslee, 1989). Findings from these studies support the validity of the PTSD diagnosis and indicate that a child is more likely to develop PTSD if the traumatic event results in physical harm to the child or in injury or death of a significant other.

Recently, clinical investigators have also begun to examine PTSD associated with sexual victimization in childhood. The purpose of this chapter is to provide information regarding the diagnosis of PTSD in sexually abused children, and to describe assessment and treatment procedures that are useful in working with child sexual abuse (CSA) survivors. Clinicians treating such children also need knowledge and skills in several other areas, including PTSD in general, PTSD in children, dynamics and sequelae of CSA, treatment strategies for young children, and cognitive–behavioral therapy.

PTSD in Child Sexual Assault Survivors

Child sexual assault is a societal problem of significant magnitude. Estimates suggest that between 150,000 and 200,000 new cases of CSA are reported each year (Finkelhor, Hotaling, Lewis, & Smith, 1984). Prevalence rates obtained from studies of adults indicate that as many as one in three women (Saunders, Villeponteaux, Lipovsky, Kilpatrick, & Veronen, in press) and one in six men (Finkelhor et al., 1984) have experienced sexual abuse in childhood.

Studies of adults who were sexually assaulted in childhood reveal striking levels of mental health problems, including depression, anxiety disorders, substance abuse, suicidality, sexual dysfunctions, and interpersonal difficulties (Lipovsky & Kilpatrick, in press). Studies examining short-term effects of CSA in children indicate that symptoms of depression and anxiety are common (Browne & Finkelhor, 1986). Many of the symptoms reported by sexually abused children or their parental figures can be understood within a PTSD framework (e.g., Goodwin, 1985). Other symptoms include sexualized behaviors, nightmares, social withdrawal or isolation, sleep difficulties, anger or acting out, somatic difficulties, and school difficulties (e.g., Adams-Tucker, 1982; Friedrich, Beilke, & Urquiza, 1988; Kolko, Moser, & Weldy, 1988).

Studies that have specifically assessed subjects for PTSD symptoms have varied widely in both their methods and their disorder prevalence rates. Estimates of the prevalence of PTSD in survivors of CSA range from 21% (Deblinger, McLeer, Atkins, Ralphe, & Foa, 1989) to 100% (Frederick, 1985). Discrepancies in PTSD rates reported in studies of children may be attributable to the use of unvalidated methods for establishing PTSD diagnostic status. Therefore, it is difficult to compare the results of these studies.

Currently, published studies of PTSD in child survivors of CSA have utilized samples referred largely from governmental agencies concerned with protective services. These studies may overrepresent cases of severe abuse, producing inflated estimates of the prevalence of PTSD. Thus, findings from these studies may not be applicable for the broader population of sexually abused children. Moreover, children whose CSA has been identified by means other than voluntary self-disclosure may be different from other sexually abused children. To date, there have been no empirical studies examining differences between children who had and had not disclosed abuse previously, or between children who disclosed abuse as a result of being asked about it in a screening or evaluation procedure and children who revealed it spontaneously. Since studies of adults abused in childhood show that only a minority ever reported their experiences to authorities (Saunders et al., in press; Finkelhor et al., 1984), it is possible that the samples studied to date may not represent the entire population of victims. However, even when their methodological weaknesses are taken into account, the results of these studies consistently show that a proportion of CSA survivors do develop symptoms reflecting PTSD.

The practical implication for clinical practice is that screening for CSA is essential in settings where children not previously identified as victims are referred because of behavioral or emotional problems. Clinicians need to be sensitive to the "at-risk" status for PTSD that these children present. In such cases, a diagnostic assessment for PTSD needs to be conducted by asking children and their parents specific questions regarding PTSD symptoms.

Theoretical Conceptualization of PTSD Associated with Child Sexual Assault

The conceptual framework that my colleagues and I use in the assessment and treatment of CSA relies upon a model used by Veronen and Kilpatrick (1980) to describe the emotional effects of rape on adult women. These authors suggest that the development of rape-related fear and anxiety can be explained by a classical conditioning model. Whereas intrusive symptoms are thought to be a function of classical conditioning, avoidance responses can be explained using an operant model (Deblinger, McLeer, & Henry, 1990). Avoidance behaviors are reinforced by the reduction in anxiety that is achieved by moving away (either physically or psychologically) from distressing cues. Additional behaviors, such as inappropriate sexual behaviors, dissociative responses, and the development of a secretive interpersonal style, may develop as a result of operant conditioning (Berliner & Wheeler, 1987).

Many potential factors involved in the conditioning process in sexually abused children may contribute to the development of emotional difficulties. Wolfe and Wolfe (1988) emphasize that multiple factors present prior to disclosure, during the disclosure phase, and following disclosure during a recovery phase may affect a child's adjustment to the sexual abuse. Friedrich (1990) also uses a multifactorial model to explain the impact of CSA. As yet, there are few research findings to reveal predictable relationships between the host of potential contributing factors and the development of PTSD. At present, then, we hypothesize that there is a relationship between the characteristics of CSA and risk for PTSD. Examples of these factors are the chronicity of the abuse, the relationship between abuser and abused, the nature of the abuse (e.g., penetration vs. no penetration), the developmental level of the child, and the reactions of others to disclosure. In the cognitive realm, a child's perception of the abuse; the meaning ascribed by the child to the abuse; and the child's thoughts about himself or herself, relationships, and the world are also hypothesized to be important factors in the development of PTSD.

Given that sexual abuse of children takes many forms and occurs in a variety of different contexts, it is not surprising that studies of the impact of CSA on children have identified a host of emotional effects. Furthermore, since much sexual abuse does not involve overtly violent or terrifying events, PTSD may not be the primary reaction for many abused children. A number of cognitive and affective issues that are often relevant to the treatment of abused children have been identified. Finkelhor (Finkelhor & Browne, 1985) has described four traumagenic dynamics of CSA: traumatic sexualization, betrayal, stigmatization, and powerlessness. These dynamics are thought to underlie psychological and behavioral effects of CSA. Finkelhor suggests that this model may explain the effects of CSA more accurately than a PTSD model. However, it may be that the persisting feelings and cognitive effects associated with these dynamics contribute to the intrusive thoughts and avoidance seen in children who develop PTSD after CSA.

Assessment

Assessing Sexual Trauma Exposure

The first step in assessment of PTSD is the identification of experiences that would qualify for the PTSD diagnosis. The severity and extent of emotional disruption in many such victims strongly suggest that CSA is an appropriate extreme stressor for the diagnosis.

Controversies related to the identification of CSA complicate the picture and contribute to the difficulties in assessment of PTSD in children. "Validating" sexual abuse becomes an issue in many cases of suspected abuse, since offenders frequently deny the allegations. However, a clinician needs to determine the likelihood that a child has experienced CSA in order to make the diagnosis of PTSD. It may be difficult to verify reported abuse experiences, because they often occur in secret and because children's disclosures are not always taken at face value by nonoffending parents or officials in the legal system. Historically, there has been profound denial on a societal level regarding the abuse of children (Summit, 1988). Nevertheless, a substantial literature exists, within which there appears to be a consensus that children rarely make up stories of sexual abuse (Wolfe & Wolfe, 1988; Faller, 1984). Although mental health professionals need to be aware of legal considerations when evaluating suspected abuse, they should not allow these to compromise their clinical approach to diagnosing PTSD.

When evaluating a child who has presented with symptoms that include externalizing (e.g., aggressive, delinquent, disruptive), internalizing (e.g., excessive crying, clinginess, social withdrawal, regression, self-destructive, nightmares), or sexualized behaviors, the clinician should be alert for the possibility of CSA. Information needs to be elicited on factors that are associated with the symptom picture. If the child does not spontaneously report uncomfortable or frightening experiences, the clinician should begin by asking open-ended questions focused on uncomfortable situations and move on to more specific questions about sexual touching.

Clinicians may be somewhat hesitant to discuss the possibility of CSA with children, out of concern that such questions may be uncomfortable to the children. It is useful to preface questions regarding possible abuse with provision of information to a child, as in the following example:

> Sometimes things happen to children [teens] that are scary or make them sad or unhappy. These are things that do not happen to most people, but when they do happen they can be very upsetting. Many times when things like this happen, children [teens] do not want to tell anybody or are afraid to tell anybody, because they don't know what will happen or because they have been told something bad might happen if they do tell. But until somebody knows what is happening, nothing can be done to stop it from happening. I am going to ask you about some things that we have found to be scary or upsetting to children [teens] and would like you to tell me

if they have ever happened to you. If you tell me about somebody touching you in a bad way or hurting you, I may have to tell other people so that we can try to make it stop. You may have to choose whether you want to answer some of these questions. I would encourage you to tell me if something is going on, so we can try to help you while you are in the hospital.

In determining whether a child has been sexually abused, somewhat different procedures may be used, depending upon the age of the child (Wolfe & Wolfe, 1988; Adams-Tucker, 1984). Older children are more likely to be responsive to direct questioning, carried out in a sensitive and supportive manner. Younger children present a more complicated picture when it comes to both assessment and treatment. Their cognitive-developmental level and mode of symptom presentation may affect the degree to which they can respond to questions regarding sexual abuse. Young children often communicate well via nonverbal, play-oriented modes. Directing children's play and eliciting drawings from them can be very useful as approaches to obtaining information regarding possible abuse (Adams-Tucker, 1984; Pynoos & Eth, 1986). In addition, anatomical dolls can be helpful to children when they relate their abuse experiences.

Although controversy exists in the CSA field in relation to the use of anatomical dolls, evidence suggests that the dolls are not likely to induce children to make false reports of abuse (Boat & Everson, 1990). Anatomical dolls are beneficial because they reduce the need for children to use language. The dolls should be presented to a child in a matter-of-fact fashion. The child should be asked to name body parts, including both sexual and nonsexual anatomy, so that the clinician is familiar with the child's names for these parts. The child can then be directed to show the clinician what he or she has experienced. The clinician should use the child's terminology throughout the evaluation (Mac-Farlane & Krebs, 1986). In addition, the clinician should not take the child's interactions with the dolls at face value, but rather should ask clarifying questions about these interactions. It is important (for legal purposes) to have some confirmation from the child that the events he or she is enacting with the dolls bear a relation to the child's own experiences.

Assessment of the trauma includes inquiry about threats or coercions utilized by the offender, the child's feelings about having disclosed, and the child's perception of how others have responded to the disclosure. Fears and concerns about these issues should be confronted directly (MacFarlane & Krebs, 1986). In addition, the specific characteristics of the child's experiences should be assessed. For example, studies of adult rape survivors suggest that cognitive perceptions are implicated in the development of PTSD. Specifically, whether the survivors believed they would be killed or seriously injured during the assault has been found to be associated with the development of PTSD (Kilpatrick et al., 1989).

In evaluating the nature of the trauma, the clinician must be sensitive to the balance between obtaining information and providing a therapeutic environment. The demands of the child protective and legal systems often create pressure for determining what happened to children as quickly as possible. However, children's fears and avoidance may inhibit them from disclosing details of their experiences, making it difficult to provide protection for them. Clinicians must often establish a buffer between these systems and the children in order to facilitate eventual complete disclosure, as well as improvements in functioning. They may need to act as advocates for these children, in order to obtain a safe place in which the children may feel able to disclose.

Assessing Symptoms of PTSD

The symptoms of PTSD can be assessed directly through questioning of the child or observation of the child's play. In addition, parent reports can be obtained. Table 6.1 provides examples of PTSD symptoms identified by each of these methods.

A supplement or "module" for assessing PTSD in children is available for the Diagnostic Interview Schedule for Children (PTSD Supplemental Module for the DISC-2.1; Fisher & Kranzler, 1990). However, psychometric properties have not been published for the DISC-2.1. Furthermore, the screening questions utilized to identify the traumatic event are limited and do not probe specifically for CSA. Therefore, many cases of CSA might well be excluded from assessment of PTSD symptomatology. Although interviews are still in the early stages of development, they constitute an important element of diagnostic measurement and merits increased use.

In the absence of validated interview schedules for children, researchers have utilized DSM-III-R criteria directly or have developed their own interviews or checklists to assess PTSD (Saigh, 1987a; McLeer, Deblinger, Atkins, Foa, & Ralphe, 1988). However, psychometric properties have not been published for any of these scales. The Impact of Event Scale (Horowitz, Wilner, & Alvarez, 1979), which was

TABLE 6.1.   Child PTSD Symptoms by Modality

Symptom	Self-report	Parent report	Child's behavior
Intrusive, repetitive symptoms	Thinks about abuse "all the time"	Child wakes with nightmares	Play with traumatic themes
Avoidance	Does not discuss abuse	Child remains isolated from peers	Child moves away from interviewer or changes activity when abuse is brought up
Hyperarousal	Reports sleep difficulties	Child reports sleep difficulties	Changes in breathing in response to questions about abuse

developed for use with adults, has been used in two studies with traumatized children (Malmquist, 1986; Yule & Williams, 1990) and appears to be useful as a quick screening measure of intrusive and avoidance symptoms. It does not, however, assess symptoms of hyperarousal, nor has it been adequately validated for use with children. One additional measure currently being validated is the Children's Impact of Traumatic Events Scale—Revised (CITES-R; Wolfe, Wolfe, Gentile, & LaRose, 1989), which includes scales measuring intrusive thoughts, avoidance, and hyperarousal to provide information about PTSD symptoms. The measure is a useful screening device for PTSD, and further evaluation may establish acceptable sensitivity and specificity for its use as a primary diagnostic test.

Existing assessment measures for use with children rely heavily upon verbal report for information gathering. However, young children in particular may not be able to describe their thoughts, feelings, and behavior, as noted earlier. Therefore, it may be necessary to include nonverbal approaches that are consistent with a particular child's developmental abilities. Pynoos and Eth (1986) have described an approach to assessing child witnesses that utilizes the children's drawings and stories about the drawings to understand their reactions to their traumatic experience. Observation of children's play (Terr, 1979; Pynoos & Eth, 1986) also provides information about their response to trauma. Although the reliability of such observational approaches to assessment has yet to be determined, such nonverbal techniques that are consistent with a child's level of development provide valuable information. Furthermore, these strategies are the only direct assessment approaches that may be feasible with very young children. Evidence for intrusive symptoms includes drawings and repetitive play involving traumatic themes. Avoidant responses can be identified when children are unable to engage in activities that remind them of the trauma. Similarly, avoidance coping may be inferred when superficial or "happy" themes predominate in the play of traumatized children.

In addition to direct assessment of a child, it is important to gather information from a parent or guardian who is familiar with the child's behavior. The Pynoos et al. (1987) reaction index has a form for use with parents in order to assess their perceptions of their children's reactions to traumatic events. In addition, Wolfe, Gentile, and Wolfe (1989) have identified items on the parent-completed Child Behavior Checklist (CBCL; Achenbach & Edelbrock, 1983) that reflect post-traumatic symptomatology.

Clinicians should note that in studies of children's responses to trauma, parents' reports tend to underestimate children's distress as compared with the children's reports (e.g., Earls et al., 1988). Conversely, studies of children's responses to CSA have consistently found greater behavioral disturbance as reported by the parents, compared with self-reported emotional difficulties of the children (e.g., Lipovsky, Saunders, & Murphy, 1989). This is a provocative area for which further research is needed to examine relationships between parent and child reports of traumatic symptoms.

Approaches to assessment of PTSD symptomatology in children are in their infancy. The coming years will probably witness growing sophistication with respect to this disorder. At present, it is recommended that researchers continue their efforts to validate and improve the measures and observational approaches that currently exist.

Additional Targets for Assessment with Sexually Abused Children

EMOTIONAL SYMPTOMS

A number of very important areas should be addressed in the assessment of sexually abused children, in addition to PTSD symptomatology. Generalized fears, anxiety, and depression have all been noted in victims of CSA (e.g., Browne & Finkelhor, 1986). Traditional measures used in practice with children include the Children's Depression Inventory (Kovacs, 1981), the Revised Children's Manifest Anxiety Scale (Reynolds & Richmond, 1978), and the State–Trait Anxiety Inventory for Children (Spielberger, 1973). Studies utilizing these self-reports measures have found that sexually abused children, as a group, do not generally score higher than the norms (Lipovsky et al., 1989; Wolfe, Gentile, & Wolfe, 1989; Mannarino & Cohen, 1986). However, scores within the normal range should not necessarily lead to the conclusion that a child has been unharmed by the abuse. It appears that traumatized children may have difficulty identifying or expressing affect with these measures. Furthermore, the measures may not relate directly to post-traumatic symptomatology.

A third self-report measure, the Fear Survey Schedule for Children—Revised (Ollendick, 1983), has been modified to include the Sexual Abuse Fear Evaluation (SAFE) subscale (Wolfe, Gentile, & Klink, 1988). Items on the SAFE reflect sex-associated fears and interpersonal discomfort.

BEHAVIORAL SYMPTOMS

The most widely used measure of children's behavioral symptoms is the parent-completed CBCL (Achenbach & Edelbrock, 1983). Sexually abused children have been found to score higher than the normative group on this measure (e.g., Mannarino & Cohen, 1986). A teacher's form of the CBCL is available and should be completed by a teacher who knows the child well. This allows the clinician to assess whether the child's maladaptive behaviors occur across situations or only in certain settings.

COGNITIVE ISSUES

Although the detrimental consequences of CSA for many children have been widely documented, it is not the case that children universally experience sexual abuse as bad, disgusting, or frightening. In many cases, abuse occurs within a context of caring and is nonviolent. Thus, it is essential that clinicians assessing sexually abused children be alert to cognitive issues related to the meaning that the abuse has for specific children. It is important that clinicians suspend their own judgments regarding children's interpretation of the abuse and work from the children's perspective.

Finkelhor's model (Finkelhor & Browne, 1985; Finkelhor, 1988) posits a number of cognitive effects of CSA. Descriptions of group treatment with child survivors generally identify an extensive list of cognitive issues that receive focus in the treatment. These include self-blame;

negative views of self, the world, and others; trust; guilt; and attributions of control. In addition, many children have learned very distorted ideas about sexuality through their experience of CSA. Cognitive factors may be associated with the development of or the exacerbation of PTSD symptoms (Powell et al., 1990). Although assessing cognitive issues in children can be difficult, the CITES-R (Wolfe, Wolfe, et al., 1989) is useful for identifying distorted cognitions about self or others, cognitions associated with Finkelhor's (1988) traumagenic dynamics, and attributional style. It is administered to the child in an interview format.

SEXUALIZED BEHAVIORS

The clinician should assess sexualized behaviors by means of the same framework as that used for assessment of other symptoms. They are included as here a separate target for assessment because (1) sexualized behaviors may be viewed as examples of intrusive thoughts being channeled into expression; (2) they are a significant component of Finkelhor's (1988) model; and (3) they are often thought to be indicators of undisclosed abuse (Berliner, Manaoia, & Monastersky, 1986). Children are often very embarrassed about their own sexual behaviors, and the clinician must be very sensitive when asking about their expression. Inquiry should be made about antecedents to sexual behaviors (e.g., "What happened before you touched Billy's peter?" "How were you feeling?"), as well as consequences (e.g., "What did your teacher do when you were touching your privates in class?"), in order to develop ideas about possible interventions. The child should be asked where she learned the behavior and what he or she is feeling before, during, and after the behaviors are enacted. In addition, parents should be asked about the frequency of sexualized behaviors and the context in which they occur (Berliner et al., 1986).

The Child Sexual Behavior Inventory (CSBI; Purcell, Beilke, & Friedrich, 1986) was recently developed to provide a systematic means of assessing children's sexual behaviors across developmental levels. Although its psychometric evaluation is incomplete, the CSBI is potentially an important instrument for providing information about the influence of CSA on the development of inappropriate sexual behaviors.

DISSOCIATIVE SYMPTOMS

Although dissociative symptoms have not been addressed widely in the CSA literature, such symptomatology in adult survivors of abuse has been discussed (Chu & Dill, 1990; Briere & Conte, 1989). In addition, a recent study (Sanders & Giolas, 1991) suggests that dissociative symptoms are associated with traumatic experiences in adolescents. Clinical experience likewise suggests that some child survivors use dissociation as an extreme form of avoidance to cope with sexual abuse. Children may report that "everything is fine," and some may skillfully cover up their thoughts and feelings. Moreover, some children may erect a "dual reality" in which the "real" reality—that of being a victim of abuse—is masked by their "safe" or "public" reality, which they must maintain. The safe reality protects the children from being overwhelmed by negative affect and may also prevent accidental disclosure or discovery of the abuse. Dissociative symptoms appear to be related to very frightening sexual abuse that leaves a child highly fearful. A behavioral analysis of situations in which the child "spaces out," loses track of time, or appears unresponsive to external stimuli is essential in such cases.

For instance, Debbie, a 9-year-old child who reported severe, sadistic sexual abuse, presented in treatment as feeling "fine"; however, her mother reported that the child had difficulty sleeping, had frequent nightmares, and appeared to be distractible in school. During a session, Debbie suddenly became unresponsive to the therapist. This state lasted for about 10 minutes, during which time the therapist attempted to maintain contact with the child. When the child "emerged" from her trance-like state, she reported that "nothing" had just happened. Upon further questioning, the child revealed that something the therapist had said reminded her of a scary part of the abuse.

Behavioral Analysis of Symptoms

If Mowrer's (1960) two-factor model of the development of PTSD is assumed, then it is essential that clinicians determine antecedents and consequences to symptoms. Although the establishment of the diagnosis requires only evidence of the specific symptoms, appropriate treatment is facilitated by knowing the pattern of symptoms, identifying salient cues that may trigger responses, and discovering contingencies that maintain those responses. Children do not always link their anxiety or avoidant symptoms to the abuse or aspects of the abuse and may report only generalized anxiety. A careful assessment can aid in establishing these links, which are important to the treatment process.

For example, Nancy reported increased anxiety related to her abusive experiences, but was unable to tie her feelings to specific aspects of the abuse. Nancy was unable to identify specific times during the day that were more distressing than others. She was asked to monitor her feelings over the following week. During the next session, Nancy indicated that she was very uncomfortable in the bathroom, particularly when she had to take a shower. Further discussion revealed that Nancy's father had surprised her in the shower on several occasions, and, although he was no longer living at home, she continued to feel anxious when showering. Specific interventions were introduced: placing a lock on the bathroom door, getting a mirror that could be placed so Nancy could see the door from within the shower, and cognitive work that helped her to use self-statements reminding her that her father was not living in the home. A decrease in anxiety symptoms surrounding showering was noted over the subsequent weeks.

Treatment

Although controlled studies of treatment for sexually abused children are lacking, the literature does already provide some guidance for the treatment of PTSD in such children. For example, a recent report by Deblinger et al. (1990) is very useful in outlining cognitive–behavioral techniques for treating child survivors of CSA. The present description of treatment approaches integrates anecdotal reports, reports of treatment of adult sexual assault survivors, and my own clinical experience. Although the potential value of group therapy with children is acknowledged, an individual approach to treatment is described.

Several general objectives guide treatment for child survivors. First, therapy is designed to help children to understand the nature of the trauma they have experienced and the effects that this experience has had on them. Second, treatment approaches should facilitate children's ability to talk and think about the abuse without embarrassment or significant anxiety. Third, intrusive, avoidant, and hyperarousal symptoms should be reduced in intensity and frequency. Finally, distorted or faulty cognitions should be altered.

Treatment should be directive, centering on the abuse itself. A therapist guides a child in examining abuse-related issues, while maintaining a supportive stance toward the child. This focus allows for emotional and cognitive processing of the abuse and its effects on the child. In addition, the therapist must take an individualized approach to setting goals and addressing important issues. Therapists working with children must always be respectful of their clients' needs for safety, and they must be willing to alter therapeutic focus or pace if children are unable to tolerate the intensity of treatment.

Facilitating Therapy

It is essential that the clinician working with a sexually abused child be very straightforward in describing the purposes of treatment. The child should be told that treatment is designed to assist him or her in coping with an event or a series of events that may be troubling, and that it is not part of an investigation (Jones, 1988). It is important that the clinician not presume that the child is distressed by the sexual abuse. In some cases, the abuse may have occurred within a context of caring and nurturance, and the child may be more distressed by separation from the family or by other people's perceptions of the implications of the abuse.

It is helpful for both clinicians and children to view the therapeutic process as one of collaboration or teamwork. Children bring their experiences, feelings, thoughts, and behaviors to the therapeutic situation, and therapists bring theoretical and technical expertise, caring, and warmth. Children are often relieved to learn that a therapist knows that talking about sexual abuse is difficult. Reassurance emphasizing that a child has choices regarding the pace and goals of treatment goes a long way toward reducing anxiety about the treatment process. It may be necessary to reorient the child to the purposes and goals of therapy at various times during the treatment process. This is especially important if the child is not participating fully in the process.

Education

Education is a primary component of therapeutic work with sexually abused children that occurs throughout the course of treatment. Children can benefit from discussions that educate them about their symptoms, about sexual issues in general, and about CSA in particular. In addition, it is helpful to describe learning principles to help in explaining how the children's symptoms may have developed and to "normalize" some of these behaviors as being predictable, given their experience of CSA. Children are often comforted by the fact that their thoughts or feelings are understandable to the therapist and that he or she has known other children who have experienced similar thoughts or feelings. Parents also can profit from information about the development of postabuse symptomatology.

Often, a child who has been chronically abused has developed a limited set of coping behaviors; in the case of a child with PTSD, these have not been effective in mediating symptoms. In addition to learning about the development of symptoms, abused children can benefit from education focused on the development of other coping strategies. Rehearsing these new skills, with feedback on performance both within and outside of the therapy session, will be an integral part of the process.

Child survivors of CSA should be provided with accurate information about sexuality, sexual development, and normal sexual behavior. Such children often develop inaccurate beliefs about sexual issues as a result of their abusive experience. Books or other published materials are helpful adjuncts for educating children about their bodies.

Group treatment provides an excellent forum for educating child survivors about abuse-related issues. Through the process of observation and discussion, each child is able to see that other children experience similar thoughts and feelings associated with their abuse. Many of the descriptions of group treatment approaches found in the literature emphasize education of children regarding specific abuse-related topics (Berliner & Ernst, 1984; Corder, Haizlip, & DeBoer, 1990; Pescosolido & Petrella, 1986).

Providing a Safe Place

As mentioned earlier, a clinician must always be sensitive to issues of safety when working with sexually abused children (e.g., MacFarlane & Krebs, 1986; Everstine & Everstine, 1989). It is useful to remember that these children have been cajoled, coerced, forced, or threatened into performing or experiencing certain behaviors that may have been frightening or uncomfortable to them. A therapeutic process that attempts to block avoidance of abuse-related issues may also be frightening or uncomfortable to the children. Therefore, a therapist must create a safe situation in which a child feels supported and has choices, as well as one that is predictable (Friedrich, 1990). Adequate orientation that attends to "ground rules" (i.e., the child does not have to talk about topics if he or she does not want to; there will be no violence or sexual touching within the therapy situation; and confidentiality is ensured) goes a long way in establishing a safe therapeutic environment. Provision of safety encourages a child to address difficult issues, despite anxiety (Pynoos & Eth, 1986). The therapist needs to gauge each child's tolerance for both psychological and physical closeness and maintain boundaries that are respectful to the child.

For example, Mary, a 10-year-old child, had been severely sexually abused by her father. She was difficult to engage in treatment and was highly avoidant of discussing issues related to the abuse. When the therapist pressed her to talk about what had happened to her, Mary became quite upset and stated, "I'm not going to do anything that I don't want to do, even if you tell me it's for my own good." Accordingly, the therapist provided Mary with a rationale for therapy and consistently inquired about the abuse, but did not require that Mary examine her thoughts and feelings about the abuse until the child indicated readiness. The therapist commented that Mary might have been frightened that the therapist would use information against her or that she might not understand Mary's feelings. She reiterated to the child that the purpose of treatment was to help her to cope with what had happened, but that they would work together at a slow and steady pace.

An approach that respects a child's need for boundaries can be very effective in empowering the child. If the child is able to take some control over the therapeutic situation by defining boundaries, he or she can potentially develop trust in the therapeutic relationship. In contrast, if the therapist ignores the child's request for space, the child is not likely to develop sufficient comfort or confidence in the therapy and may not be capable of moving forward in a healthy manner. One must remember, however, that therapy has a purpose, and the child should be reminded of this frequently. The therapist should consistently inquire about issues and communicate to the child that it is important to discuss feelings and the abuse, while also being mindful of the child's ability to tolerate the intensity of the process. The therapist should not allow the child's avoidance to completely block therapeutic focus on the trauma. Discussion of reasons for avoidance and interpretations regarding the process of treatment can help get the child back on track.

In addition to issues related to psychological safety, sexually abused children often express significant concerns regarding physical safety in the therapeutic setting. For instance, James was a 7-year-old child who had been forced to fondle his father's genitals. His father had warned him that he always knew where James was and whom he was talking to. Even though James's father now lived in another state, James constantly feared that his father knew what he was saying to the therapist during treatment sessions. In the first several sessions, James asked the therapist whether she was recording their discussions. Although she reassured him that she was not, James looked under the desk and in drawers to ensure that there was no tape recorder on. This activity became a ritual that began each therapy session. The ritual was maintained for several months until after James disclosed details of the abuse and received support from his therapist.

The therapist must do whatever is necessary and reasonable to promote the child's sense of safety. It is often helpful to remind the child that he or she has survived the initial disclosure and that the offender's threats have not been carried out. Unfortunately, it is not always the case that the child may be protected from some of the feared consequences of disclosure. The therapist, working within a community intervention system, should function as an advocate to minimize the chances that the child will experience negative repercussions for disclosing.

Allowing Affective Expression

A significant proportion of therapy with CSA survivors is directed toward the expression of affect (e.g., Sturkie, 1983; Salter, 1988). Encouraging affective release within a safe and supportive environment enables the child to experience feelings without the need for avoidance. Throughout treatment, the child will be encouraged and assisted in recognizing and labeling feelings associated with the abuse. This process should occur throughout treatment whenever new issues or memories are brought up.

A frequent symptom of PTSD is "numbing" or restricted range of feelings. As noted earlier, children may indicate that they feel "nothing," that they are "fine," or that they "don't know" how they are feeling. It seems that these children may have needed to dissociate thoughts from feelings during abusive episodes in order to cope with overwhelming negative affect. However, this defensive style may generalize to nonabusive but emotionally distressing situations, and the children may not learn to identify feelings accurately or express them appropriately. If a child is unable or unwilling to explore affective responses to CSA, it may be helpful to approach other, less threatening topics that may provide a forum for affective expression. Drawings, storytelling, and the use of puppets are helpful media that allow the child to explore affective issues at a distance.

For example, JoAnne, a 12-year-old who was abused by her father over a period of 3 years, was reluctant to disclose details of the abuse in treatment and generally indicated that she was "fine." However, her mother reported that JoAnne had difficulty sleeping and was socially withdrawn. Since she enjoyed drawing pictures, she was directed to draw a picture of a girl. JoAnne was then asked a number of questions about the girl's likes and dislikes, things that made the girl feel certain ways, and things the girl did when she felt certain ways. She was able to identify the girl's feelings in relation to everyday types of events. When JoAnne was asked how the girl might react to more distressing situations, the drawing technique was used to assist her in identifying feelings that the girl in the picture might have in response to a number of different situations. JoAnne improved in her ability to recognize the range of the girl's responses, and she began to acknowledge that she too had a variety of feelings.

Use of Developmentally Appropriate Techniques

Although even young children are capable of engaging in some elements of "talk" therapy, there are many other avenues available to facilitate the processing of abuse-related material. Therapists need to be flexible in the use of a variety of techniques that reduce the demand on children to utilize language for expression. In addition, a child's need to control distress levels by "distancing" from uncomfortable topics needs to be respected.

PLAY

Children often communicate through play as an alternative to direct verbal communication. Play is a useful medium for sexually abused children to play out traumatic themes, fears, and distorted beliefs (e.g., Walker & Bolkovatz, 1988; Marvasti, 1989). Repetitive trauma-related play is noted in the DSM-III-R as a re-experiencing phenomenon that may be seen in children with PTSD (American Psychiatric Association, 1987).

Play provides an opportunity for children to process thoughts and feelings associated with abuse in symbolic as well as direct ways (Walker & Bolkovatz, 1988). It is often less threatening to children than direct verbal interaction, because it allows for some distance between the children and the scenes they are enacting. However, Terr (1981) has suggested that traumatic play may not extinguish by itself and should not automatically be viewed as an adaptive coping mechanism in children. She suggests that it is often necessary for such play eventually to be interrupted in order for a child to begin to heal from the trauma. Furthermore, when the therapist is able to join in the play with the child, repetitive patterns suggestive of re-experiencing symptoms can be changed into new positive methods of coping without the need for extensive explanation.

For instance, Jason, a 4-year-old child, had been sexually abused by his father. In addition, his father had coerced several children in the neighborhood into participating in the abuse. Although Jason could provide little detail regarding the abuse, it was suspected that several of the abuse incidents were quite violent. In his play, Jason repetitively enacted scenes in which a small doll was pursued and physically assaulted by a larger doll. The small doll appeared unable to escape from these assaults. The therapist introduced another large doll into the play. This "rescuer" was positioned between the "victim" and "pursuer" dolls. The "rescuer" stated, "Stay away from Jason. I will not let you hurt him." Blocking the repetition of Jason's play allowed him to enact approach behaviors of the "victim" toward the "rescuer." Jason's anxiety appeared to decrease somewhat, and he was able to give an identity to the "rescuer" and to reveal his perceptions of the responses of others to his disclosure. Blocking the repetitive play appeared to free Jason up to explore other issues and concerns, both through play and through direct verbal disclosure of additional details of the abuse.

Play also has a distracting function and can be useful in working with older children from this perspective. Often, therapy sessions may proceed while a therapist and child are playing checkers or cards. This process helps to minimize the child's anxiety while difficult issues are being discussed, through distracting the child from the source of the anxiety. Several therapeutic games are also useful for approaching difficult subject areas and addressing distorted beliefs. The "Talking, Feeling, and Doing Game" (1973) and the "Rainbow Game" (1989) are two such games that encourage the child to express feelings, enact situations behaviorally, and discuss difficult topics.

DRAWINGS

The value of drawings cannot be underestimated in work with children. They provide an opportunity for a child to communicate about issues from a distance, and they can serve as a medium for therapeutic manipulation of events. Berliner's (1987) work in this area has been instructive.

Karen, for example, had been abused by her stepfather. Although he was no longer living in the home, she reported having dreams in which he was chasing her around the house. She was asked to draw a picture of that scene. In addition, she and the therapist worked to draw another picture to make the scene less frightening. In this revised picture, the stepfather tripped over a piece of furniture; Karen pushed him out of the house and locked the door. Karen was instructed to remember this ending for the scene if the nightmare should return.

ROLE PLAYING

Role playing is useful in helping the child to enact more adaptive behaviors, particularly those related to self-protection. Mitchell, for instance, had been sexually assaulted by his baseball coach. Within the therapy, several potentially dangerous scenarios were described, and Mitchell was helped to enact behaviors to protect himself. He practiced saying, "Go away from me; I will tell if you do something wrong," when the therapist took on the aggressive role.

Role playing can facilitate the identification of distorted beliefs or maladaptive responses. Utilizing role reversal with traumatized children can be a valuable approach to revealing their beliefs about the thoughts and feelings of others. Using puppets as characters in role-play enactments allows the children to address important issues while maintaining a degree of psychological distance.

STORIES

Therapeutic stories also have considerable value in the treatment of sexually abused children. They can present traumatic issues, describe alternative coping methods, or link important feelings or behaviors to abusive situations. Davis and Sparks (1988) have compiled a useful collection of stories that focus on a variety of themes relevant to abused children. In addition, many books written specifically for children describe other children's reactions and experiences related to sexual abuse.

Therapists should utilize their own creativity in devising stories that reflect particularly salient issues for individual children. In particular, metaphors can be useful for illustrating important themes for older children and adolescents. For example, Tammy, a 16-year-old who had been abused by her grandfather, was experiencing significant fear, anxiety, and depression that she had difficulty expressing. The therapist utilized the metaphor of sitting on a garbage can to keep all the "junk" (i.e., bad feelings, frightening thoughts) from coming out. She noted to Tammy that sitting on this garbage can greatly limited her ability to move about and experience her world, and that the "junk" was leaking out anyway. Tammy was encouraged to jump off the can, let the junk out, recycle what could be recycled, throw the unneeded garbage out, and put the rest back in the can. In this way, the can could be emptied a bit and she would not have to sit on it to keep the junk down. This metaphor was utilized throughout treatment when Tammy attempted to avoid examination of important therapeutic material.

DIARIES AND SELF-MONITORING

Many children as young as 8 can monitor events, thoughts, and feelings that occur between sessions. Self-monitoring facilitates the identification of links between traumatic events and current behavioral or emotional functioning. Monitoring can be accomplished through the use of diaries, particularly with older children. Writing in the diary can also provide a coping mechanism for dealing with intrusive thoughts, particularly when they are bothersome at times when talking with others may be impractical (e.g., at night). Children should be instructed to write down their thoughts and feelings if they are having difficulty getting them out of their minds. Diary materials can be brought to the therapy session to be used as the focus of intervention, or children may keep their diaries to themselves as a private record of thoughts and feelings.

Strategies for Coping with Anxiety

Before initiating approaches that involve exposure, a clinician will find it helpful to teach a child several strategies for coping with anxiety. Appropriate use of these techniques can facilitate the child's sense of control over his or her feelings. In addition, the techniques can be used in conjunction with exposure procedures to protect the child from becoming overwhelmed by negative affect.

DEEP MUSCLE RELAXATION

Deep muscle relaxation is used in systematic desensitization, but it also is a useful procedure in its own right. The goal is to teach the child a practical way to reduce fear and anxiety. Ollendick and Cerny (1981) provide detailed instructions on training procedures. This training is quite useful to children outside the therapy room when they find themselves in anxiety-producing situations.

Steven, for example, was to testify in court about his sexually abusive experiences. He was quite anxious about having to see the offender in the courtroom and was uncomfortable talking about the abuse. He was instructed in the use of deep muscle relaxation and cue-controlled breathing. During his testimony, Steven became nervous when asked specific questions about the abuse. He began to use the cue-controlled breathing technique and was able to continue his testimony. Following his appearance in court, Steven reported to the therapist that breathing and telling himself to relax helped him to concentrate on the questions without worrying about his own fear.

Although most children appear to enjoy the relaxation and breathing exercises once they overcome initial uneasiness, abused children can experience heightened anxiety at the prospect of letting down their guard. In particular, children may be reluctant to close their eyes to complete the procedure. In such a case, the therapist should explore with the child the meaning of "relaxing." Some children will state that they do not want to relax because they will then not be ready if something "bad" were to happen. Reassurance by the therapist regarding safety in the session is often sufficient to overcome a child's reluctance. In addition, the therapist can keep the duration of the exercise brief or begin the relaxation and breathing exercises while the child keeps his or her eyes open. Successive approximations may be necessary so that the child is eventually able to relax with eyes closed throughout the complete procedure.

Children can be instructed to practice the relaxation procedures at home during quiet times and to use them in "scary" situations. Relaxation procedures can also be utilized in conjunction with abuse-focused discussions or at the end of therapy sessions to reduce a child's level of tension.

DISTRACTION TECHNIQUES

Distraction techniques are also useful tools for controlling anxiety. Since PTSD often involves significant avoidance symptoms, many sexually abused children may already be proficient in the use of distraction as a defense against experiencing affect. However, distraction in therapy is used not to block feelings, but as a tool for coping with anxiety engendered by abuse-focused sessions. When distraction is used in this way, a child can experience negative affect without losing control. Positive imagery, particularly having the child imagine a "safe place" as mentioned earlier, can provide relief from anxiety. In addition, having the child discuss difficult issues while playing cards, checkers, or drawing can help to offset anxious feelings. As relaxation procedures do, this process provides the child with a concrete set of behaviors that can be utilized to cope with anxiety.

Roberta, a 10-year-old abused by her uncle, was taken through the relaxation procedures described above. Then she was directed to imagine a place where she could feel safe. She was asked to describe this place in great detail. Following several sessions in which this guided imagery was practiced, Roberta was encouraged to begin discussing specific abusive experiences. When the therapist observed Roberta becoming upset, she directed the child to imagine her safe place. Such imagery was utilized for several minutes to allow Roberta to calm herself somewhat, and the exploration of the abuse events was resumed. Roberta was able to continue to focus on the abuse itself, with several short periods of using guided imagery to keep her anxiety at a manageable level.

Exposure Techniques

The cornerstone of treatment with a sexually abused child is a direct focus on the abuse experiences themselves (Corder et al., 1990; Deblinger et al., 1990; Friedrich, 1990; Berliner & Ernst, 1984). These techniques encourage the child to approach uncomfortable memories, thoughts, discussions, and feelings in the absence of objective threat (Deblinger et al., 1990). The immediate goal is to reduce or extinguish the child's arousal, in a safe environment, in response to abuse-related stimuli. Subsequently, avoidance may be reduced so that the child is able to think, feel, and talk about the abuse without becoming too uncomfortable.

Exposure techniques have several additional benefits. First, discussion of actual abuse experience helps to reveal cues present during the abuse itself that may have taken on significance as conditioned stimuli for activating anxiety. Important reinforcement contingencies can be identified when retelling the story allows the therapist to evaluate the dynamics of the child's experience. Second, exposure techniques encourage the experience and expression of affect. Affect can be labeled, and its meaning can be explored. Finally, the therapist's knowledge of the specifics of the abuse can facilitate the clarification of maladaptive cognitions.

Exposure can be accomplished in a variety of ways, and the approach used should be developmentally appropriate. Whereas most children above the age of 6 or 7 can talk about important issues, dolls, drawings, storytelling, letter writing, and diaries are useful exposure techniques with younger children. Adolescents should be encouraged to write down their trauma-related thoughts and feelings when these occur outside of the therapy session.

SYSTEMATIC DESENSITIZATION

Systematic desensitization has been used widely in the treatment of anxiety disorders in both children and adults (Ollendick & Cerny, 1981). Anxiety-producing scenes are presented imaginally to a child while he or she is in a state of deep muscle relaxation. The child is involved in the development of the scene hierarchy which proceeds from those that are mildly upsetting to those that elicit maximal distress. Desensitization presents graduated exposure to traumatic memories under the assumption that anxiety and relaxation are incompatible responses. Thus, the child's painful anxiety associated with recalling the abuse will be reduced.

An informal, less structured, and more naturally occurring process is recommended for desensitization therapy a child. Inquiries are made of the child regarding abuse-related issues. When a situation or issue is identified that the child is able to tolerate discussing, it should become the focus of the treatment. If the child begins to experience an increase in anxiety, the relaxation response can be induced, and the child can be guided to explore the issue further. As the child approaches more and more difficult issues, he or she learns that the relaxation response can be used to cope with discomforting affect.

FLOODING

Flooding procedures (Stampfl & Levis, 1967) are used under the assumption that extinction of traumatic emotional responses will occur when the child re-experiences the traumatic event in a safe setting. Accordingly, repeated imaginal presentations of the traumatic scenes are made. The procedure includes attention to sensory cues (e.g., odors, sounds) within the imagined scene, and cognitive interpretations and attributions related to the scene. Flooding has been used in a systematic fashion by Saigh (1987b) to treat war-traumatized children, and in a less structured manner by Pynoos and Eth (1986) with children exposed to violence. The procedure is appropriate for a sexually abused child, provided that the therapist takes care to ensure that the child is not overwhelmed by affective responses. It is likely to be most successful if the child is allowed some choices, if the exposure periods are kept to a relatively brief period of time (e.g., 15 minutes), and if the relaxation procedure is used at the end of the flooding session.

It is recommended that clinicians working with child survivors of CSA utilize an approach that incorporates elements from both systematic desensitization and flooding. In this combined approach, a child is asked to address abuse-related memories, thoughts, and issues, and is encouraged to re-experience the affects associated with these stimuli as in the flooding procedure. Although the child is encouraged to experience as much affect as possible, relaxation and distraction approaches are utilized to prevent the child from becoming overwhelmed. Also unlike flooding, this approach proceeds from mildly through more intensely distressing issues, rather than focusing on the most distressing issues first.

The process of repeated disclosure and exploration occurring in a safe, supportive environment can work to counteract avoidance and denial, and allows the child to experience thoughts and feelings without automatically denying them or dissociating from them. The child needs to be able to tolerate exposure to memories of the abusive experiences, in order to explore and ultimately integrate them in an adaptive manner. It is important that the therapist assist each child in finding the "therapeutic window" (Cole & Barney, 1987), which is the psychological area between being overwhelmed by thoughts or feelings and being cut off from feelings. The most successful treatment probably occurs at the juncture at which the child is experiencing a moderate level, of distress such that he or she is motivated by the discomfort but is not prevented from exploring discomforting memories by overwhelming affect.

Cognitive Approaches

Maintaining a focus on abuse-related issues provides a context within which cognitive therapeutic interventions can be utilized. The goals of cognitive work with sexually abused children are (1) to provide children with additional coping techniques to deal with anxiety; (2) to correct faulty or irrational thinking; and (3) to clarify the basis of beliefs regarding the meaning of the abuse (Berliner & Wheeler, 1987). The primary techniques that can be utilized with these children include thought stopping, guided self-dialogue, and cognitive restructuring.

THOUGHT STOPPING

Thought stopping is a relatively simple procedure first described by Wolpe (1958) that has been used in the treatment of adult rape survivors (Veronen & Kilpatrick, 1983). Thought stopping is utilized to interrupt ruminative thinking. The child is instructed to think about abuse-related issues, and then the therapist says "Stop!" in a loud voice. The therapist should then check to be sure that the statement has effectively interrupted the child's thoughts. Then the child is instructed to practice saying "Stop!" aloud when he or she notices repetitive, persistent thoughts. When the child is able to do this successfully, he or she is instructed to say "Stop!" silently. An alternate procedure is to have the child wear a rubber band around his or her wrist and to snap it and say "Stop!" silently when intrusive thoughts arise.

GUIDED SELF-DIALOGUE

Guided self-dialogue or mediated self-talk is often useful as an anxiety reduction strategy with sexually abused children (Deblinger et al., 1990). In addition, this cognitive strategy can be an important component of skills training and intervention with sexually inappropriate behaviors. The approach is modeled after a procedure described by Meichenbaum (1977).

Exploration of a child's self-statements may often reveal that they are negative, exacerbate anxiety, and foster an avoidant response. For instance, Timmy was extremely avoidant of abuse-related issues in therapy; although several approaches were attempted, he remained unable to address important topics. The therapist began exploring the reasons for the avoidance, and Timmy stated, "I cannot handle talking about it because I get so upset I can't think straight." The assumption is that such negative self-statements are maladaptive, and the goal is to replace these with other, more self-enhancing statements. Guided self-dialogue, therefore, involves identifying irrational, faulty, or negative self-statements and teaching the child to replace these with rational, positive statements. Timmy was taught relaxation and guided imagery procedures to facilitate coping with anxiety. He was praised for the skills he had acquired and was told that these strategies would be able to assist him in situations that were frightening. Negative self-statements he made about inability to manage abuse-related feelings were challenged, and within the session positive self-statements were generated and practiced out loud. Timmy was able to state, "I now know some ways to help myself if I get upset. I know that [my therapist] will also help me to not get too afraid. I can discuss the abuse without falling apart. We will take it one step at a time, and I will use what I have learned to help myself get over this." After practicing these statements aloud, Timmy was encouraged to say them silently to himself. He was also directed to pay attention to negative self-statements used in situations other than the therapy sessions, to try to turn them into positive statements, and to bring these up in future sessions. Thus, the strategy learned for coping with abuse-related discussions was generalized to other anxiety-producing circumstances.

COGNITIVE RESTRUCTURING

Cognitive restructuring requires an exploration of the child's belief systems and cognitive misinterpretations. The goal is to provide alternative cognitions that are more accurate and adaptive. The procedure can be thought of as an extension of guided self-dialogue. It is a more complex process than merely replacing one set of cognitions with another, because it involves more in-depth exploration of the source of faulty cognitions before more adaptive cognitions can be substituted (McCann, Pearlman, Sakheim, & Abrahamson, 1988). This process is utilized because it is believed that unhealthy cognitions may be a component of what underlies the intrusion–avoidance pattern.

An issue that can serve as an example for describing cognitive restructuring is the sense of self-blame that child victims frequently express. In the past, clinical lore suggested that children needed only to be reassured that the abuse was not their fault and that they were not responsible. However, it is also essential to explore the underlying beliefs that contribute to children's assumption of responsibility and help the children to see for themselves that they were not at fault.

Hannah, for instance, had been abused by her father for several years. She stated to her therapist, "I know you are telling me the truth when you say the abuse was not my fault. I know it in my head, but sometimes I just don't believe it. If I was not wrong for being abused, then I would have told someone about it to make it stop." The therapist explored the reasons why Hannah did not disclose the abuse. The child noted that at various times her father had told her that he would go to jail, that her mother would not believe her, and that the family would fall apart if she told anyone about the abuse. The therapist assured Hannah that she understood that these were frightening consequences, and that she had made a choice not to disclose because she thought that disclosing would make things worse. The therapist stated that Hannah should not have had to make that choice, but that her father put her in the position of having to choose between a number of scary choices. Hannah was also helped to see that her choice not to disclose was made so that she could protect her family; it was not evidence that the abuse was her fault.

This example serves to illustrate that cognitive restructuring is a complicated process. Children must examine their own beliefs about themselves, the abuse, and other people, and therapists must provide clarifying information as well as opportunities for the children to challenge their own beliefs. In Hannah's case, her father did go to jail. Although she had done well with restructuring beliefs about her responsibility for the abuse, she then presented the view that it was her fault that her father had gone to jail, because "he told me he would if I let anyone know about the abuse." Hannah was asked what she would do if she saw someone rob a bank. "I would tell the police," she said. She was asked what she would do if a stranger did what her father did to her. "I would tell my mother." The therapist then asked Hannah to think about what made the current situation different. "He is my father," she replied. Additional exploration was conducted to ascertain what this meant to her. Although Hannah appeared to understand cognitively that she had done nothing wrong by disclosing, she continued to experience somewhat negative feelings about the consequences of the disclosure. Further clarification was necessary to help Hannah to see that her father had gone to jail because of what he did rather than because she disclosed abuse.

Targets for cognitive restructuring are identified by careful assessment, particularly of the issues identified by Finkelhor (1988) and Porter, Blick, and Sgroi (1982). Betrayal, powerlessness, stigmatization, guilt, and trust are particularly important issues to be approached with a cognitive restructuring strategy. Furthermore, over the course of treatment additional faulty cognitions will be identified.

Cognitive restructuring can be difficult to accomplish at times. First, a child's avoidance to exploring abuse-related thoughts must be overcome to some degree, in order to be able to identify faulty cognitions. Anxiety reduction strategies and exposure techniques should be employed. Second, family dynamics and the responses of others to the child's disclosure will affect the cognitive restructuring process. It may be quite difficult to challenge the child's beliefs if these beliefs are partially supported by reality, as they were in Hannah's case.

Other Approaches to Re-Experiencing Symptoms

Re-experiencing symptoms, including intense distress at reminders of the abuse, flashbacks, hallucinations, and nightmares, are often very frightening to children and may require direct intervention. A behavioral analysis that identifies the context in which intrusive symptoms occur, the content of the symptoms, and possible reinforcing contingencies should be conducted. Examination of the context in which intrusive symptoms occur can identify their relationship to abuse-related stimuli. Education regarding conditioning processes and direction in the use of relaxation, distraction, and/or cognitive procedures are used to intervene.

Steven, a 12-year-old who had been molested by a neighbor, reported feeling panicky when getting off the school bus in the afternoons. He could not readily identify anything that reminded him of the abuse in this situation. However, when discussing the abuse, Steven noted that the neighbor had sometimes driven by when Steven was walking home from the bus stop. Together, the therapist and Steven were able to determine that his anxiety was in anticipation of seeing the neighbor (who actually was in jail). Steven was taught to use the relaxation response and to repeat positive self-statements (i.e., "Mr. Z is not around. He will not drive by. Even if he does, he will not hurt me again").

A useful approach to nightmares and flashbacks is to assist the child in changing their content (Berliner & Wheeler, 1987). After the child describes the content of the nightmare, the therapist and child focus on facilitating the development of an alternative ending to the scenario or an alternative response that may be used within the scenario. The alternative response may be developed using guided imagery, drawing, or play. This procedure helps to interrupt the re-experiencing cycle, and also provides the child with a coping response to address future intrusive symptoms.

Skills Training

Excellent descriptions of skills training procedures that are useful with children can be found in Ollendick and Cerny (1981). Assertiveness training and social skills training have important roles in the treatment of sexually abused children (Corder et al., 1990; Sturkie, 1983). They can have the effect of increasing the children's sense of self-efficacy, can provide them with strategies for protecting themselves from further abuse, and can increase their sense of self-confidence.

Skills training should involve a detailed behavioral assessment of a child's skill deficits and inappropriate behaviors developed as adaptations to abuse (Sturkie, 1983). Cognitions related to self-efficacy also may require a restructuring approach before the child is able to benefit from skills training. Alternatively, skills training may provide the child with evidence of his or her ability to succeed or to have control in a situation, which can then be used to challenge faulty cognitions. With practice, the child should begin to feel a sense of control in previously uncomfortable situations. Positive self-statements to be used in place of negative cognitions can be generated from success experiences; this facilitates the generalization of appropriate use of skills to new situations.

Teaching a child a structured problem-solving approach can facilitate the recognition of faulty cognitions and maladaptive behaviors, so that the child can identify more adaptive means of responding. The sequence of events when the child responds in a maladaptive fashion is to (1) analyze the context in which the behavior or cognition occurred, with particular attention to potential conditioned stimuli; (2) link conditioned stimuli to cues present in the abuse situation, if possible; and (3) construct a set of choices for alternative responses in the absence of abuse.

Another approach to problem solving, described by Meichenbaum and Goodman 1971), follows this sequence: (1) What is the problem? (2) What is my plan? (3) Am I using my plan? and (4) How did I do? The final step in this sequence is very important, as it involves the development of children's ability to evaluate their own behavior accurately and to reinforce themselves for adaptive solutions to the problem.

Sexual abuse prevention can be viewed as a skill-building approach. In particular, a child is taught self-protective strategies and is helped to generate specific responses to be utilized if a potentially dangerous situation arises. Role-play rehearsal can help to offset avoidant responses by increasing the child's self-efficacy in dealings with adults (Berliner & Ernst, 1984).

Sexual abuse prevention involves educating the child about social cues, providing factual information about sexual abuse, and helping the child to differentiate types of touching (Deblinger et al., 1990). It is important to work with the child to generate and practice response strategies to be used if someone should approach him or her in an inappropriate way. However, it is also important to discuss the possibility that an adult might succeed in perpetrating abuse even if the child should utilize a protective strategy, so that if the strategy fails, the child does not feel that he or she is a failure or is to blame. It is useful to point out the size and power differential that existed during the abusive events the child has already experienced, and to let the child know that sometimes using appropriate self-protective strategies is not sufficient to prevent abuse from occurring. A problem-solving approach should be utilized to generate possible responses to such a situation.

Dealing with Sexually Inappropriate Behaviors

Current research suggests that child victims may exhibit more sexualized behaviors than normals (Friedrich et al., 1987), as noted earlier. The strategies described for dealing with victimization-related re-experiencing and avoidance symptoms may also help reduce sexual acting out (Johnson & Berry, 1989; Berliner et al., 1986). The focus should be on education regarding normative sexual behaviors; expression of feelings associated with the child's sexual behaviors (both antecedent and consequent feelings); utilization of anxiety reduction strategies if anxiety stimulates the child's sexual arousal; social skills training; and cognitive restructuring procedures that replace inappropriate thinking and disinhibiting self-statements with rational thoughts and self-controlling statements. A careful analysis of the antecedents and consequences of the sexualized behavior, the meaning that it has for the child, and the thoughts and feelings associated with the behavior is necessary.

Involving Parents in Treatment

Since our model of PTSD includes an operant component, whereby avoidance behaviors are maintained by consequences in a child's environment, aspects of the environment require examination. In particular, the responses of nonoffending parents and perpetrators to children's disclosures may have a tremendous impact on whether the children are able to address issues related to the abuse during the recovery process. Children's reactions to the abuse, their willingness to share with a therapist, and their tolerance for examining their feelings about the abuse will all be affected by the manner in which parents cope with events. Parents may benefit from their own individual therapy, particularly nonoffending parents who themselves may have been abused. In particular, parents' involvement with their children about issues related to the abuse is important to address.

Parents, as well as children, can benefit from education regarding the effects of sexual abuse (Conte & Berliner, 1988; Everstine & Everstine, 1989). Parents can begin to understand their children's emotional, cognitive, and behavioral difficulties if they are exposed to the theoretical models used by the therapist to explain the development of these difficulties. Involving parents in individual sessions focused on their feelings about the abuse and their expectations of their children is useful as a graduated exposure approach to their own reactions, so that they are better able to help their children cope with the victimization (Deblinger et al., 1990).

Parents may be used to intervene directly with their children by teaching them traditional behavior management techniques (see Ollendick & Cerny, 1981). Parents can be instructed to use positive reinforcement, redirection of the children's behavior, and time out as appropriate to intervene with maladaptive behaviors. Parents can reinforce the appropriate use and practice of anxiety reduction techniques. Finally, parents provide valuable information based upon their observations of their children outside of the therapy situation. Therefore, parents may be asked to monitor behaviors and report the frequency of occurrence, as well as the context in which the behaviors occur.

Termination

Treatment may be appropriately terminated when a child's intrusive, avoidant, and hyperarousal symptoms decrease to a level that does not interfere with adaptive functioning. The child should be able to discuss abuse-related issues with minimal emotional discomfort, should not be displaying sexualized behavior, and should have a clear sense of the fact that he or she was not at fault within the abusive situation. The therapist may predict potentially difficult situations in the future (e.g., onset of puberty, development of more intimate relationships) that may be associated with a recurrence of symptomatology. The child and parents should be encouraged to seek therapeutic assistance if symptoms should recur.

Impediments to Treatment

Although treatment may be unsuccessful for many reasons, three are somewhat specific to work with children who have developed PTSD as a result of CSA. First, a child's avoidance symptoms, which are a target of treatment, can be formidable obstacles to engaging the child in exposure techniques. The therapist must explore this process with the child.

For example, Larry, a 12-year-old who had been assaulted by a 19-year-old boy in the neighborhood, had been involved in exposure techniques for several months of treatment. He came in to his session one day and stated that he had to talk about something but did not want to. He and the therapist discussed his reluctance, but did not get far. The therapist asked Larry whether he was afraid that the material he needed to talk about would cause the therapist to think badly of him. Larry said that he was afraid that the therapist would think Larry had wanted the abuse to happen after the therapist heard what he had to say. The therapist reassured Larry that he knew Larry was upset about the abuse and that the older boy was at fault. Larry slowly began to discuss his concerns about his own sexual response to the abuse. This was a very significant issue that would have been missed if the therapist had not been able to overcome Larry's avoidance.

A second frequent impediment to treatment is the response of authorities to a child's disclosure. Uncertainty about visitation, discomfort with investigators and legal professionals, and ambivalence about consequences to the offender can exacerbate the child's distress. The therapist may need to be more active in cases of abuse than in other types of cases, to ensure that the systems and individuals dealing with the needs of the child have up-to-date information and are working toward solutions that are in the child's best interests.

Finally, therapists themselves can be impediments to treatment. Therapists must be comfortable dealing with sexual issues and need to be able to tolerate listening to very unpleasant topics without becoming overly distressed in the presence of children. Knowledge and skills are needed in normal child development, child psychopathology, abuse-related issues, legal considerations related to CSA, and therapeutic techniques. Therapists treating victimized children need to maintain a collegial network of others professionals who can be consulted on a regular or emergency basis for input on specific cases. In addition, the network provides a necessary source of emotional support by those who are knowledgeable about issues related to treatment of sexually abused children. These are essential safeguards for trauma therapists to reduce the risk of professional "burnout."

References

Achenbach, T. M., & Edelbrock, C. (1983). *Manual for the Child Behavior Checklist and Child Behavior Profile.* Burlington: University of Vermont, Department of Psychiatry.

Adams-Tucker, C. (1982). Proximate effects of sexual abuse in childhood: A report on 28 children. *American Journal of Psychiatry, 139,* 1252–1256.

Adams-Tucker, C. (1984). Early treatment of child incest victims. *American Journal of Psychotherapy, 38,* 505–516.

American Psychiatric Association. (1987). *Diagnostic and statistical manual of mental disorders* (3rd ed., rev.). Washington, DC: Author.

Arroyo, W., & Eth, S. (1985). Children traumatized by Central American warfare. In S. Eth & R. S. Pynoos (Eds.), *Post-traumatic stress disorder in children* (pp. 103–120). Washington, DC: American Psychiatric Press.

Berliner, L. (1987). *Assessment and treatment of child victims of sexual abuse.* Workshop presented at the Medical University of South Carolina, Charleston.

Berliner, L., & Ernst, E. (1984). Group work with preadolescent sexual assault victims. In I. Stuart & J. G. Greer (Eds.), *Victims of sexual aggression: Men, women, and children* (pp. 105–124). New York: Van Nostrand Reinhold.

Berliner, L., Manaoia, O., & Monastersky, C. (1986). *Child sexual behavior disturbance: An assessment and treatment model.* Unpublished manuscript.

Berliner, L., & Wheeler, J. R. (1987). Treating the effects of sexual abuse on children. *Journal of Interpersonal Violence, 2,* 415–434.

Bloch, D. A., Silber, E., & Perry, S. E. (1956). Some factors in the emotional reaction of children to disaster. *American Journal of Psychiatry, 113,* 416–422.

Boat, B. W., & Everson, M. D. (1990). When the tail wags the dog: The response to legal challenges of the credibility of children's allegations of sexual abuse. *Child, Youth and Family Services Quarterly, 13,* 2–3.

Briere, J., & Conte, J. (1989, August). *Amnesia in women molested as children: Testing theories of repression.* Paper presented at the annual meeting of the American Psychological Association, New Orleans.

Browne, A., & Finkelhor, D. (1986). Impact of child sexual abuse: A review of the research. *Psychological Bulletin, 99,* 66–77.

Burke, J. D., Borus, J. F., Burns, B. J., Millstein, K. H., & Beasley, M. C. (1982). Changes in children's behavior after a natural disaster. *American Journal of Psychiatry, 139,* 1010–1014.

Chu, J. A., & Dill, D. L. (1990). Dissociative symptoms in relation to childhood physical and sexual abuse. *American Journal of Psychiatry, 147,* 887–892.

Cole, C. H., & Barney, E. E. (1987). Safeguards and the therapeutic window: A group treatment strategy for adult incest survivors. *American Journal of Orthopsychiatry, 57,* 601–609.

Conte, J., & Berliner, L. (1988). The impact of sexual abuse on children: The empirical findings. In L. E. A. Walker (Ed.), *Handbook on sexual abuse of children: Assessment and treatment issues* (pp. 72–93). New York: Springer.

Corder, B. F., Haizlip, T., & DeBoer, P. (1990). A pilot study for a structured, time-limited therapy group for sexually abused pre-adolescent children. *Child Abuse and Neglect, 14,* 243–251.

Davis, N., & Sparks, T. (1988). *Therapeutic stories to heal children* (rev. ed.). Oxon Hill, MD: Psychological Associates.

Deblinger, E., McLeer, S.V., Atkins, M., Ralphe, D., & Foa, E. (1989). Post-traumatic stress in sexually abused children, physically abused, and non-abused children. *Child Abuse and Neglect, 13,* 403–408.

Deblinger, E., McLeer, S. V., & Henry, D. (1990). Cognitive behavioral treatment for sexually abused children suffering post-traumatic stress: Preliminary findings. *Journal of the American Academy of Child and Adolescent Psychiatry, 29,* 747–752.

Dollinger, S. J., O'Donnell, J. P., & Staley, A. A. (1984). Lightning-strike disaster: Effects on children's fears and worries. *Journal of Consulting and Clinical Psychology, 52,* 1028–1038.

Earls, F., Smith, E., Reich, W., & Jung, K. G. (1988). Investigating psychopathological consequences of a disaster in children: A pilot study incorporating a structure diagnostic interview. *Journal of the American Academy of Child and Adolescent Psychiatry, 27*, 90–95.

Everstine, D. S., & Everstine, L. (1989). *Sexual trauma in children and adolescents: Dynamics and treatment.* New York: Brunner/Mazel.

Faller, K. C. (1984). Is the child victim of sexual abuse telling the truth? *Child Abuse and Neglect, 8*, 473–481.

Finkelhor, D. (1988). The trauma of child sexual abuse: Two models. *Journal of Interpersonal Violence, 2*, 348–366.

Finkelhor, D., & Browne, A. (1985). The traumatic impact of child sexual abuse: A conceptualization. *American Journal of Orthopsychiatry, 55*, 530–541.

Finkelhor, D., Hotaling, G., Lewis, I. A., & Smith, C. (1984). Sexual abuse in a national survey of adult men and women: Prevalence, characteristics, and risk factors. *Child Abuse and Neglect, 14*, 19–28.

Fisher, P., & Kranzler, E. (1990). *Post-traumatic stress disorder: Supplemental module for the DISC-2.1.* New York: New York State Psychiatric Institute.

Frederick, C. J. (1985). Children traumatized by catastrophic situations. In S. Eth & R. S. Pynoos (Eds.), *Post-traumatic stress disorder in children* (pp. 71–100). Washington, DC: American Psychiatric Press.

Friedrich, W. N. (1990). *Psychotherapy for sexually abused children and their families.* New York: Norton.

Friedrich, W. N., Beilke, R. L., & Urquiza, A. J. (1987). Children from sexually abusive families: A behavioral comparison. *Journal of Interpersonal Violence, 2*, 391–402.

Goodwin, J. (1985). Post-traumatic stress symptoms in incest victims. In S. Eth & R. S. Pynoos (Eds.), *Post-traumatic stress disorder in children* (pp. 157–168). Washington, DC: American Psychiatric Press.

Handford, H. A., Mayes, S. D., Mattison, R. E., Humphrey, F. J., Bagnato, S., Bixler, E. O., & Kales, J. D. (1986). Child and parent reaction to the Three Mile Island nuclear accident. *Journal of the American Academy of Child Psychiatry, 25*, 346–356.

Horowitz, M., Wilner, N., & Alvarez, W. (1979). Impact of Event Scale: A measure of subjective stress. *Psychosomatic Medicine, 41*, 209–218.

Johnson, T. C., & Berry, C. (1989). Children who molest: A treatment program. *Journal of Interpersonal Violence, 4*, 185–203.

Jones, D. P. H. (1986). Individual psychotherapy for the sexually abused child. *Child Abuse and Neglect, 10*, 377–385.

Kilpatrick, D. G., Saunders, B. E., Amick-McMullan, A., Best, C.L., Veronen, L.J., & Resnick, H.S. (1989). Victim and crime factors associated with the development of crime-related post-traumatic stress disorder. *Behavior Therapy, 20*, 199–214.

Kinzie, J. D., Sack, W. H., Angell, R. H., Manson, S., & Rath, B. (1986). The psychiatric effects of massive trauma on Cambodian children: I. The children. *Journal of the American Academy of Child Psychiatry, 25*, 370–376.

Kolko, D. J., Moser, J. T., & Weldy, S. R. (1988). Behavioral/emotional indicators of sexual abuse in child psychiatric inpatients: A controlled comparison with physical abuse. *Child Abuse and Neglect, 12*, 529–541.

Kovacs, M. (1981). Rating scales to assess depression in school-aged children. *Acta Paedopsychiatrica, 46*, 305–315.

Lipovsky, J. A., & Kilpatrick, D. G. (in press). The child sexual abuse victim as an adult. In W. O'Donohue & J. H. Geer (Eds.), *The sexual abuse of children: Theory, research, and therapy.* Hillsdale, NJ: Erlbaum.

Lipovsky, J. A. Saunders, B. E., & Murphy, S. M. (1989). Depression, anxiety, and behavior problems among victims of father–child sexual assault and nonabused siblings. *Journal of Interpersonal Violence, 4*, 452–468.

MacFarlane, K., & Krebs, S. (1986). Techniques for interviewing and evidence gathering. In K. MacFarlane, J. Waterman, & Assocates, *Sexual abuse of young children: Evaluation and treatment* (pp. 67–100). New York: Guilford Press.

Malmquist, C. P. (1986). Children who witness parental murder: Posttraumatic aspects. *Journal of the American Academy of Child Psychiatry, 25*, 320–325.

Mannarino, A. P., & Cohen, J. A. (1986). A clinical–demographic study of sexually abused children. *Child Abuse and Neglect, 10*, 17–23.

Marvasti, J. A. (1989). Play therapy with sexually abused children. In S. M. Sgroi (Ed.), *Vulnerable populations: Evaluation and treatment of sexually abused children and adult survivors* (Vol. 2, pp. 1–41). Lexington, MA: Lexington Books.

McCann, L., Pearlman, L. A., Sakheim, D. K., & Abrahamson, D. J. (1988). Assessment and treatment of the adult survivor of childhood sexual abuse within a schema framework. In S. M. Sgroi (Ed.), *Vulnerable populations: Evaluation and treatment of sexually abused children and adult survivors* (Vol. 1, pp. 77–101). Lexington, MA: Lexington Books.

McLeer, S. V., Deblinger, E., Atkins, M. S., Foa, E. B., & Ralphe, D. L. (1988). Posttraumatic stress disorder in sexually abused children. *Journal of the American Academy of Child and Adolescent Psychiatry, 27*, 650–654.

Meichenbaum, D. H. (1977). *Cognitive-behavior modification.* New York: Plenum.

Meichenbaum, D. H., & Goodman, J. (1971). Training impulsive children to talk to themselves: A means of developing self-control. *Journal of Abnormal Psychology, 77*, 115–126.

Mowrer, O. H. (1960). *Learning theory and behavior.* New York: Wiley.

Nader, K., Pynoos, R. S., Fairbanks, L., & Frederick, C. (1990). Children's PTSD reactions one year after a sniper attack at their school. *American Journal of Psychiatry, 147*, 1526–1530.

Ollendick, T. H. (1983). Reliability and validity of the Revised Fear Survey Schedule for Children (FSSC–R). *Behaviour Research and Therapy, 21*, 685–692.

Ollendick, T. H., & Cerny, J. A. (1981). *Clinical behavior therapy with children.* New York: Plenum.

Pescosolido, F. J., & Petrella, D. M. (1986). The development, process, and evaluation of group psychotherapy with sexually abused preschool girls. *International Journal of Group Psychotherapy, 36*, 447–469.

Porter, F., Blick, L., & Sgroi, S. (1982). Treatment of the sexually abused child. In S. Sgroi (Ed.), *Handbook of clinical intervention in child sexual abuse* (pp. 109–146). Lexington, MA: D.C. Heath.

Purcell, J., Beilke, R. L., & Friedrich, W. N. (1986, August). *The Child Sexual Behavior Inventory: Preliminary normative data.* Paper presented at the annual convention of the American Psychological Association. Washington, DC.

Pynoos, R. S., & Eth, S. (1986). Witness to violence: The child interview. *Journal of the American Academy of Child and Adolescent Psychiatry, 25*, 306–319.

Pynoos, R. S., Frederick, C., Nader, K., Arroyo, E., Steinberg, A., Eth, S., Nunez, F., & Fairbanks, L. (1987). Life threat and posttraumatic stress in school age children. *Archives of General Psychiatry, 44*, 1057–1063.

Pynoos, R. S., & Nader, K. (1988). Psychological first aid and treatment approach to children exposed to community violence: Research implications. *Journal of Traumatic Stress, 1*, 445–473.

Rainbow Game. (1989). Warner Robins, GA: Rainbow House, Children's Resources Center.

Reynolds, C. R., & Richmond, B. O. (1978). "What I Think and Feel": A revised measure of children's manifest anxiety. *Journal of Abnormal Child Psychology, 6*, 271–280.

Saigh, P. A. (1987a). In vitro flooding of an adolescent's posttraumatic stress disorder. *Journal of Clinical Child Psychology, 16*(2), 147–150.

Saigh, P. A. (1987b). *The development and validation of the Children's Posttraumatic Stress Disorder Inventory.* Paper presented at the meeting of the Association for Advancement of Behavior Therapy, Boston.

Salter, A. C. (1988). *Treating child sex offenders and victims: A practical guide.* Newbury Park, CA: Sage.

Sanders, B., & Giolas, M. H. (1991). Dissociation and childhood trauma in psychologically disturbed adolescents. *American Journal of Psychiatry, 148*, 50–54.

Saunders, B. E., Villeponteaux, L. A., Lipovsky, J. A., Kilpatrick, D. G., & Veronen, L. J. (in press). Child sexual assault as a risk factor for mental disorders among women: A community survey. *Journal of Interpersonal Violence.*

Spielberger, C. D. (1973). *Preliminary manual for the State–Trait Anxiety Inventory for Children ("How I Feel Questionnaire").* Palo Alto, CA: Consulting Psychologists Press.

Stampfl, T. G., & Levis, D. J. (1967). Essentials of implosive therapy: A learning-theory-based psychodynamic behavioral therapy. *Journal of Abnormal Psychology, 72*, 496–503.

Stoddard, F. J., Norman, D. K., & Murphy, J. M. (1989). A diagnostic outcome study of children and adolescents with severe burns. *Journal of Trauma, 29*, 471–477.

Sturkie, K. (1983). Structured group treatment for sexually abused children. *Health and Social Work, 8*, 299–308.

Summit, R. C. (1988). Hidden victims, hidden pain: Societal avoidance of child sexual abuse. In G. E. Wyatt & G. J. Powell (Eds.), *Lasting effects of child sexual abuse* (pp. 39–60). Newbury Park, CA: Sage.

Talking, Feeling, and Doing Game: A psychotherapeutic game for children. (1973). Cresskill, NJ; Creative Therapeutics.

Terr, L. C. (1979). Children of Chowchilla: A study of psychic trauma. *Psychoanalytic Study of the Child, 34*, 547–623.

Terr, L. C. (1981). "Forbidden games": Post-traumatic child's play. *Journal of the American Academy of Child Psychiatry, 20*, 741–760.

Titchener, J. L., & Kapp, F. T. (1976). Family and character change at Buffalo Creek. *American Journal of Psychiatry, 133*, 295–299.

Veronen, L. J., & Kilpatrick, D. G. (1980). Self-reported fears of rape victims: A pre-liminary investigation. *Behavior Modification, 4*, 383–396.

Veronen, L. J., & Kilpatrick, D. G. (1983). Stress management for rape victims. In D. Meichenbaum & M. Jaremko (Eds.), *Stress reduction and prevention* (pp. 341–374). New York: Plenum.

Walker, L. E. A., & Bolkovatz, M. A. (1988). Play therapy with children who have expe-rienced sexual assault. In L. E. A. Walker (Ed.), *Handbook on sexual abuse of children: Assessment and treatment issues* (pp. 249–269). New York: Springer.

Wolfe, V. V., Gentile, C., & Klink, A. (1988). *Psychometric properties of the Sexual Abuse Fear Evaluation (SAFE)*. Unpublished manuscript, University of Western Ontario.

Wolfe, V. V., Gentile, D., & Wolfe, D.A. (1989). The impact of sexual abuse on chil-dren: A PTSD formulation. *Behavior Therapy, 20*, 215–228.

Wolfe, V. V., & Wolfe, D. A. (1988). The sexually abused child. In E.J. Mash & L.G. Terdal (Eds.), *Behavioral assessment of childhood disorders* (2nd ed., pp. 670–714). New York: Guilford Press.

Wolfe, V. V., Wolfe, D. A., Gentile, C., & LaRose, L. (1989). *Children's Impact of Traumatic Events Scale—Revised*. Unpublished manuscript, University of Western Ontario.

Wolpe, J. (1958). *Psychotherapy by reciprocal inhibition*. Stanford, CA: Stanford Uni-versity Press.

Yule, W., & Williams, R. M. (1990). Post-traumatic stress reactions in children. *Journal of Traumatic Stress, 3*, 279–295.

Index

M

Malingering, 47, 48
Marital discord, skills training, 64
Marital Happiness Inventory, 18
Medical center inpatient care, 39–66
Medications (*see* Psychotropic medications)
Menlo Park Vietnam Veterans Treatment Program, 40
Military history assessment, 16, 17
MMPI
  battered women, PTSD subscale, 76
  Vietnam veteran evaluation, 18, 52
Molestation (*see* Sexual molestation)
Motivation for treatment, 23
Mowrer's two-factor theory, 49
Multidisciplinary team treatment, 41–43
Muscle relaxation (*see* Deep muscle relaxation)

N

Narcissistic personality disorder, 20, 21
Nightmares
  combat-related PTSD, 36
  sexually abused children, 155
  symptom pattern of PTSD, 6
Nonverbal assessment techniques, 134, 135
Nursing staff
  importance of cooperation of, 43
  observations of, 41
  in treatment team, 41–43

O

Operant conditioning model, 129

P

Paranoid personality disorder, 20
Partial PTSD, 10

Peer counseling
  advantages, 17
  Vietnam veterans, 13, 17, 18
Personal responsibility
  anger as undercutting factor, 29
  and healing process, veterans, 28
Personality, battered women, 80
Personality disorders
  combat-related PTSD, 20, 21, 35, 44, 46, 49, 50
  differential diagnosis, 44
  inpatient treatment, 46
Physiological arousal
  battered women, 71, 76
  combat-related PTSD, 7, 52, 53, 56
  and flooding, 56
  management of, 90
  sensitivity and specificity of assessment, 53
  sexual-assault-related PTSD, 113
  sexually abused children, 134
Play, sexually abused children, 132–134, 144, 145
Post-traumatic stress disorder (PTSD)
  conceptual model, 7–9
  epidemiology, 3–6
  symptom patterns, 6, 7
  validity of diagnosis, 2–4
Potentiation relationship, 8, 9
Pretrauma adjustment
  assessment, 51
  combat-related PTSD, 20, 44, 51
  sexual assault survivors, 104, 105
Prisoners of war, 19
Problem solving
  battered women, 85–87
  combat-related PTSD, 32
  sexually abused children, 156
Protective factors, 8
Psychiatrists, in treatment team, 41, 42
Psychological Maltreatment of Women Inventory, 75
Psychologists, in treatment team, 41
Psychopathology
  definition, 4
  epidemiology, 5, 6

Victimization, battered women, 91, 92
Vietnam veterans, 13–36
  anger as central dynamic, 28, 29
  assessment, 16–18, 49–53
  behavioral treatment, inpatients,
    53–66
  chronicity of symptoms, 35, 36
  cognitive restructuring, 60–64
  combat exposure, 5
  comorbidity, 19–21, 42–46
  compensation/pension considerations,
    47, 48
  confrontation technique, 35
  course of PTSD, 19
  crisis intervention, 21–23
  cultural rejection, 15
  early developmental trauma, 20
  family relationships, 33, 34
  flooding, inpatients, 55–60
  group therapy, 24–30
  inpatient treatment, 39–66
  motivation for treatment, 23
  and personality disorders, 20, 21, 35
  physiological assessment, 52, 53
  premilitary functioning, 44, 51
  psychopathology rates, 6
  relapse of trauma symptoms, 31
  treatment, 21–33, 39–66
  "uniformity myth," 17
  unique trauma experiences, 14–16
Vietnam Veterans History Question-
    naire, 51, 52
Vigilance, 33–35
Violence, potential for, 103, 104
Voice, 14
Vulnerability, 8, 9

W

War-related PTDS (*see* Combat trauma)
Women therapists, 93